I would like to dedicate this book to my three wonderful sons Aaron, Adam, and Aric for their support and encouragement throughout the process of writing this book. I would also like to dedicate this book to my 93-year-old mother, Fran Schmidt, who instilled in me a love of physical activity, health, and fitness at a very early age.

# Contents

# Fitness

## STEPS TO SUCCESS

Nancy L. Naternicola

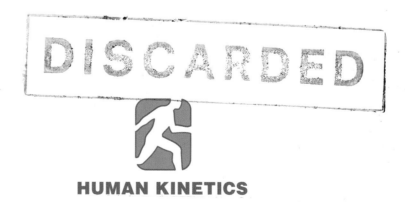

**HUMAN KINETICS**

**Library of Congress Cataloging-in-Publication Data**

Naternicola, Nancy L., 1952-

Fitness : steps to success / Nancy L. Naternicola.

   pages cm

Includes bibliographical references.

1.  Physical fitness.  I. Title.

GV481.N26 2014

613.7--dc23

                 2014019021

ISBN: 978-1-4504-6885-5 (print)

The web addresses cited in this text were current as of October 2014, unless otherwise noted.

**Acquisitions Editor:** Justin Klug and Michelle Maloney; **Developmental Editor:** Anne Hall; **Managing Editor:** Tyler M. Wolpert; **Associate Managing Editor:** Nicole Moore; **Copyeditor:** Jan Feeney; **Permissions Manager:** Martha Gullo; **Senior Graphic Designer:** Keri Evans; **Cover Designer:** Keith Blomberg; **Photographs (cover and interior):** Neil Bernstein; **Photo Asset Manager:** Laura Fitch; **Visual Production Assistant:** Joyce Brumfield; **Photo Production Manager:** Jason Allen; **Art Manager:** Kelly Hendren; **Associate Art Manager:** Alan L. Wilborn; **Illustrations:** © Human Kinetics, unless otherwise noted; **Printer:** Versa Press

We thank the West Virginia University Student Recreation Center in Morgantown, West Virginia, for assistance in providing the location for the photo shoot for this book.

Human Kinetics books are available at special discounts for bulk purchase. Special editions or book excerpts can also be created to specification. For details, contact the Special Sales Manager at Human Kinetics.

Printed in the United States of America     10 9 8 7 6 5 4 3 2 1

The paper in this book is certified under a sustainable forestry program.

**Human Kinetics**

Website: www.HumanKinetics.com

*United States:* Human Kinetics
P.O. Box 5076
Champaign, IL 61825-5076
800-747-4457
e-mail: humank@hkusa.com

*Canada:* Human Kinetics
475 Devonshire Road Unit 100
Windsor, ON N8Y 2L5
800-465-7301 (in Canada only)
e-mail: info@hkcanada.com

*Europe:* Human Kinetics
107 Bradford Road
Stanningley
Leeds LS28 6AT, United Kingdom
+44 (0) 113 255 5665
e-mail: hk@hkeurope.com

*Australia:* Human Kinetics
57A Price Avenue
Lower Mitcham, South Australia 5062
08 8372 0999
e-mail: info@hkaustralia.com

*New Zealand:* Human Kinetics
P.O. Box 80
Torrens Park, South Australia 5062
0800 222 062
e-mail: info@hknewzealand.com

E6149

# Climbing the Steps to Fitness Success

Get ready to climb a staircase—one that will lead you to become fit and more knowledgeable about the components of fitness: cardiovascular health, muscular strength and endurance, flexibility, balance, and core strength and stability. You cannot leap straight to the top, but you can reach it by climbing one step at a time.

Not many books on fitness are written so that an inexperienced person can easily understand the information and use it with confidence. Terminology is often confusing, explanations are unclear, and readers are expected to understand too much information at one time. The approach taken in this book does not assume that one explanation or illustration is enough to allow you to become knowledgeable about and skilled at developing all the components of fitness. Instead, carefully developed procedures accompany each step and provide you with ample practice and opportunities for self-assessment.

This book focuses on two primary areas. First, it helps you assess your fitness level to determine what areas of fitness you need to improve and what areas you need to maintain. Second, it provides the knowledge you need in order to design your own fitness program that will improve and maintain those areas of fitness. We begin by providing you with an overview of fitness that explains the components and exercising training principles. Next you will learn how to perform a health screening to make sure you can safely proceed to fitness testing. Included in the health self-assessment are risk factors for heart disease, pulse, blood pressure, body measurements, BMI, and girth measurements. This is followed by fitness testing that will determine baselines for cardiovascular fitness, muscular strength and endurance, flexibility, balance, and core strength. Results from these tests will help you determine if you need to improve in these areas or maintain these areas. Once you know what you need to do, you will set goals for reaching the fitness level you desire. These goals are based on your interests, schedule, lifestyle, and fitness level. Once goals are set, important information regarding each component of fitness is explained that includes the benefits and recommendations (frequency, intensity, time, and type) of the exercises. This is followed by instructions on preparing to start exercising, including selecting types of cardiorespiratory exercises, flexibility exercises, and various types of strength training exercises. Building on this foundation of information, we introduce basic exercises and follow them with descriptions of techniques specific to the exercises recommended in this book.

We have taken great care to introduce new information and higher training intensities gradually. For instance, you will start out lifting lighter training loads (weight) while you are learning proper exercise technique. Later, after you have mastered the exercises, you will progress to heavier loads. Organizing and sequencing exercises and loads in this manner offer you the best opportunity to learn how to perform the exercises without fear of injury, and will provide an excellent opportunity for you to realize dramatic improvements in muscular endurance, strength, body composition, and overall fitness. Exercises that develop a specific muscle area using body weight or exercise equipment are described. You will also incorporate balance and core training into your fitness program. After completing steps 4 through 8 on each of the five components, you will have designed your own fitness program and will be ready to begin.

You will find that the steps to performing the exercises in this text are unique and provide an effective approach to understanding the skills of each exercise. The step-by-step explanations and self-assessment activities make this book the easiest guide to fitness.

This book also includes a discussion on nutrition and using skills to eat more healthfully. This is followed by a section on behavior and recognizing your readiness to change and using strategies to change your behavior.

Each of the 10 steps you will take is an easy transition from the one that precedes it. The first 3 steps of the staircase provide a solid foundation of basic information you need in order to begin your fitness journey. As you progress, you will learn to engage in a safe and efficient fitness program. You will also learn when and how to make needed changes in program intensity. As you near the top of the staircase, you will find that you have developed a sense of confidence in exercising and knowledge of designing programs that meet your needs. Perhaps most important, you will be pleased with your improved fitness, energy level, and appearance.

The Steps to Success method is a systematic approach to executing and teaching each component of fitness. Approach each of the steps in this way:

1. Read the explanation of what is covered in the step, why the step is important, and how to execute the tasks described in each step; these may be a basic skill, a concept, an approach, or combination of all three.

2. Follow the technique photos that show exactly how to position your body so that you will perform each exercise correctly. The photos show each phase of the exercise. Look over the missteps section after each exercise description and use this information to make needed corrections in performing the exercises.

3. At the end of each step, read the Success Summary and answer the review questions to make sure you are ready to move to the next step.

After you have selected an intensity level and time in step 4 for cardiorespiratory exercise, you are ready to choose a strength exercise for each body area in step 5 and a flexibility exercise for each body area in step 6. You will then add step 7, balance, and step 8, core, to your fitness program. The instructions, as well as examples and self-assessment opportunities, will prepare you for the challenge of designing your own program. Good luck on your step-by-step journey toward developing a strong, healthy, attractive body. It's a journey that will be confidence building, rich in successes, and fun!

# Acknowledgments

I would like to thank several people at Human Kinetics who influenced the development and completion of this book. Justin Klug, Michelle Maloney, Anne Hall, Neil Bernstein, and Martha Gullo. I would also like to thank my wonderful, talented models Kara Myers, Brendan Marinelli, Eric Dunbar, Emily Gardner, Calvin Moore, Sarah Cover, Hope Sloanhoffer, Kaylea Dulaney, and Greg Thomas.

# Overview of Fitness

I f I asked you what the word *fitness* means to you, how would you answer? Different people have different definitions. Does it mean being thin or having a specific body type? Or eating healthfully and not using harmful substances such as tobacco or drugs? Does it mean regularly working out at the gym? In fact, all these definitions are correct. Total fitness is a state of health that includes weight management, muscular strength, and good nutrition.

If you consider regular exercise a component of physical fitness, you will get even more definitions. To one person, muscular strength might mean weightlifting, while to another it might mean being able to run 10 miles. But today when we talk about physical fitness, we refer to five distinct areas that should be included: cardio, resistance training, flexibility, balance, and core training. Each of these areas should be included in *everyone's* workout program! In this book we explain all of these components and why they are important. We also demonstrate how to measure each component so you are able to design a workout program that will maintain the areas in which you rated average or better and improve the areas in which you rated below average or poor.

## SUCCESS CHECK

- ☒ What is meant by fitness?
- ☒ What are the five components of physical fitness?

# COMPONENTS OF FITNESS

Each of the five areas of physical fitness plays an important role in being fit, and one is not more important than another. Think about the components of a car: What's the use in having a nice-looking exterior if the motor is shot or the tires are flat? In comparison, weightlifters may have nice physiques but not be able to run a mile; runners may complete a mile in record time but not be able to complete a push-up.

# Cardiorespiratory Fitness

Cardiorespiratory fitness is how efficiently your heart and lungs are able to deliver oxygen to the working muscle, which means it has a direct impact on both strength and endurance. The heart is a muscle and must be worked to be strong and efficient just as other muscles of the body. Not only is cardio the base for all activity, but keeping your heart in good condition also helps prevent many health problems. Following are more benefits from having a healthy heart:

- Adds years to your life
- Increases the HDL (good) cholesterol in the body
- Decreases the LDL (bad) cholesterol in the body
- Lowers blood pressure
- Lowers resting pulse so your heart doesn't have to work as hard
- Helps you lose or maintain weight
- Helps prevent heart disease and stroke
- Lowers your risk for developing diabetes
- Reduces stress levels
- Boosts your immune system
- Increases energy
- Improves sleep

### SUCCESS CHECK

- ☒ What is cardiorespiratory fitness?
- ☒ Name five benefits of cardiorespiratory fitness.

# Resistance Training

Resistance training involves challenging your muscles to work against an external force in order to improve endurance, increase muscle mass, and improve strength. It is imperative to include resistance training in your workout plan because strong muscles make strong tendons, which make strong and dense bones. This in turn reduces the risk of osteoporosis.

After age 20, adults lose five to seven pounds of muscle every decade. Resistance training will help stop this loss of muscle and rebuild the muscle at *any* age! Muscle is *active* tissue, so you must use it or you will lose it. Having strong, toned muscles improves your ability to perform everyday activities, including getting in and out of the bathtub and carrying grocery bags. There are many other benefits of resistance training:

- Helps control weight (increases calorie burn)
- Improves balance and decreases risk of injury
- Reduces low back pain
- Boosts stamina
- Reduces blood pressure
- Increases metabolism

- Maintains or increases joint flexibility
- Helps reduce pain from arthritis
- Improves insulin sensitivity and glucose metabolism
- Reduces depression
- Improves brain function
- Enhances appearance

### SUCCESS CHECK

- ☒ What is resistance training?
- ☒ Why is it important to include resistance training in your workout?

# Flexibility

Flexibility is the range of motion around a joint. It is the cornerstone of your workout program because your muscles move only as far as your flexibility allows. Tight joints restrict range of motion, causing you to compensate the movement by using other muscles. This can cause muscle imbalances that affect posture, performance, and movement efficiency. Loss of flexibility can also lead to lost independence; for example, you can no longer bend to clip your toenails or reach the high shelf in your kitchen.

Incorporating flexibility into your workout (at any age) can improve posture and make movement more efficient. It also aids in these areas:

- Reduces back pain
- Improves digestion
- Enhances performance
- Decreases the risk of injury
- Improves muscular coordination
- Enhances circulation

### SUCCESS CHECK

- ☒ What is flexibility?
- ☒ Why is it important?

# Balance

Balance is the ability to control your body's position in space. It involves proprioception, which is how your body takes the information it receives from the environment (such as getting up from a chair) and sends this information to the brain. This information tells the muscles what to do so they can adapt to the change and you keep your balance. When this system gets overloaded, you lose your balance. Whether you are standing still (static balance) or moving (dynamic balance), your body continually makes adjustments to keep you from falling. Although you may think that having good balance is important only for gymnasts or figure skaters, regular balance training improves posture and coordination, enhances movement and performance, and helps prevent injuries and falls.

## Core Strength and Stability

Core muscles are responsible for extending, flexing, and rotating your trunk. These consist of many layers of muscle that will determine your posture. Strengthening and conditioning these muscles reduce the chances of back pain and spinal injuries, improve performance, and result in better coordination and balance. Therefore, all exercise programs should consist of a solid foundation of core work.

# WHY GETTING BASELINE MEASUREMENTS IS IMPORTANT

Without knowing where you stand, how do you know what direction to go? Baseline measurements are the road map to your fitness program. By completing baseline measurements composed of a health screening and fitness tests, not only will you know where you stand but you will also know what to include in your fitness program to improve or maintain your fitness level. Do you need to strengthen or stretch specific muscle groups for better posture or performance? Improve balance? What changes do you need to make in your body composition (fat mass versus fat-free mass) to be within healthy guidelines? At what intensity level should you start in the areas of cardio, muscle, or flexibility?

More important, baseline measurements function as a screening tool that indicates whether you need a physician's referral before starting an exercise program. It also brings to light any exercise that may be contraindicated for you. In addition, baseline measurements allow you to track progress. It can be used as a motivational tool as well as a factor in setting goals. These measurements are simple and can be done in the privacy of your own home. Although some of the tests may call for assistance from a friend or family member, such as girth measurements and posture checks, you can complete most of these by yourself. You can perform a balance test, flexibility measurement, or push-up test in your living room. No need to be frightened about a test—remember that you are just gathering information to make educated decisions for your workout that will be beneficial for your health, time, and fitness level.

# FITTE PRINCIPLE

Each of the five components of fitness has a set of rules that you must follow in order for you to gain any benefit from your exercise program. The FITTE principle is an acronym of these rules. You can use these principles to establish guidelines in designing a workout program for your individual needs and fitness level. In addition, these guidelines will help you set goals and design a plan that fits your schedule. It will also help you get past plateaus in weight loss and prevent boredom.

## Frequency

Frequency means the number of times a week you need to perform the exercise as seen in table 1.1. Keep in mind that these are guidelines and may have to be modified according to your baseline results, and each component has its own set of guidelines.

Table 1.1    Required Frequency for Various Types of Exercise

| Cardio | |
| --- | --- |
| **Proficiency** | **Frequency** |
| Moderate (40-60% of maximum heart rate) | 5 days/week |
| Vigorous (>60% of maximum heart rate) | 3 days/week |
| Combination of moderate/vigorous | 3-5 days/week |
| **Resistance training** | |
| **Proficiency** | **Frequency** |
| Beginner or not currently training | 2-3 days/week |
| Intermediate | 3-4 days/week |
| Advanced | 4-5 days/week |
| **Flexibility** | |
| **Proficiency** | **Frequency** |
| Minimum | 2-3 days/week |
| Preferred | 5-6 days/week |
| **Balance** | |
| **Proficiency** | **Frequency** |
| Beginner | 3 days/week |
| Intermediate/Advanced | 2-3 days/week |

*(continued)*

**Table 1.1** *(continued)*

| Core strength and stability | |
|---|---|
| **Proficiency** | **Frequency** |
| Beginner/Intermediate/Advanced | 2-3 days/week |

Sources: American College of Sports Medicine, 2010, *ACSM's guidelines for exercise testing and prescription,* 8th ed. (Philadelphia: Wolters Kluwer), 153 (cardio), 173 (flexibility); T.R. Baechle, R.W. Earle, and D. Wathen, 2008, Resistance training. In *Essentials of strength training and conditioning,* 3rd ed., edited for the National Strength and Conditioning Association by T.R. Baechle and R.W. Earle (Champaign, IL: Human Kinetics), 389 (resistance training); Canadian Fitness Professionals, 2012, *Foundations of professional personal training* (Champaign, IL: Human Kinetics), 54 (flexibility); V.H. Heyward and A.L. Gibson, 2014, *Advanced fitness assessment and exercise prescription,* 7th ed. (Champaign, IL: Human Kinetics), 353 (balance); Human Kinetics, 2010, *Core assessment and training* (Champaign, IL: Human Kinetics) (core).

# Intensity

Intensity is one of the most important as well as one of the most complicated factors in the FITTE principle because measuring intensity in a cardio workout is different than measuring intensity in a resistance training workout as shown in tables 1.2 (instructions for performing the talk test and RPE can be found in Step 4) and 1.3. Improvements in your fitness level will be impaired if you are not working out at the proper intensity level.

## Table 1.2   Evaluating Intensity for Cardio

| Cardio activity level | Fitness class | Intensity MHR | Talk test | RPE 0-10 |
|---|---|---|---|---|
| Sedentary: extremely deconditioned | Poor | 30-45% | | 1-2 |
| Minimal activity: moderate to high deconditioned | Poor/ fair | 40-55% | | 3 |
| Sporadic physical activity: moderate to mild deconditioned | Fair/ average | 55-70% | | 4-5 |
| Habitual physical activity: moderate to vigorous exercise | Average/ good | 65-80% | | 6-7 |
| High amounts of habitual activity: vigorous exercise | Good/ excellent | 70-85% | | 8-9 |

Table 1.3   Optimal Intensity for Resistance, Balance, Core Strength, and Flexibility

| Resistance, balance, and core strength | | |
| --- | --- | --- |
| Training goal | Sets | Repetitions |
| General fitness | 1-2 Sets | 8-15 Reps |
| Muscular endurance | 2-3 Sets | >12 Reps |
| Muscular hypertrophy | 3-6 Sets | 6-12 Reps |
| Muscular strength | 2-6 Sets | < 6 Reps |
| Flexibility | | |
| Flexibility | To the point of tension, not pain. | |

Adapted, by permission, from T.R. Baechle, R.W. Earle, and D. Wathen, 2008, Resistance training. In *Essentials of strength training and conditioning*, 3rd ed., edited for the National Strength and Conditioning Association by T.R. Baechle and R.W. Earle (Champaign, IL: Human Kinetics), 406; W.L. Westcott, 2003, *Building strength and stamina*, 2nd ed. (Champaign, IL: Human Kinetics).

## Time

Time is how long each session should last, and it is unique for each fitness component. According to ACSM guidelines, a cardio workout can last anywhere from 10 to 60 minutes depending on intensity levels.

Resistance training is much more complicated when it comes to time because it depends on the type of program you are doing. A circuit of 8 to 10 weight training machines consisting of a single set can take as little as 15 minutes, whereas a split routine with multiple exercises and sets per muscle group can take up to 45 minutes.

When it comes to stretching, ACSM guidelines state the stretch should be held for 10 to 30 seconds. Holding a stretch longer than 30 seconds causes the muscle to start contracting as the result of your body's stretch reflex.

Balance training and core training are included in the resistance portion of your workout and follow the same guidelines.

## Type

Today there are many types of exercise options available that were nonexistent 10 years ago. You do not need to join a fitness facility to design and implement a complete fitness program, nor do you need expensive fitness equipment.

Cardio exercises can be done at a gym, outdoors in your neighborhood, or in your living room. These include traditional treadmill, stepper, or other fitness machine, group fitness classes, running, boxing, and sports such as basketball and racquetball.

Resistance training has also evolved over the past few years. Instead of the traditional choice of free weights or machines, you have the option of boot camp classes, kettlebells, TRX training, and DVDs (P90X and Insanity) or on-demand fitness in your living room.

The flexibility component has also evolved over time. We now see mind–body classes and more emphasis on mobility and stretching than in the past. Your flexibility workout should include all the major muscle groups with special attention paid to areas that are tight. Major muscles include the large muscles of the body such as quads, glutes, back, and chest. Tight areas in most individuals are hamstrings, low back, chest, and calves.

## Enjoyment

The final component that has been added in recent years is *enjoyment*! If you do not find joy in what you are doing, you will not see long-term success. Enjoying what you do will help you adhere to your exercise program and keep you motivated.

### SUCCESS CHECK

- ☒ What does the acronym FITTE stand for?
- ☒ Name some of the new exercise options available today.

# PRINCIPLES OF EXERCISE TRAINING

To better design and implement a fitness program, you need to understand principles of exercise training. This will guide you in the FITTE principles. Principles of exercise training are specificity, reversibility, overload, and progression.

## Specificity

The principle of specificity states that doing specific training or activity will produce specific results. For example, if you want to get stronger, you need a resistance program. If you want to run, you must follow a running program. If you want to be better at tennis, you must practice tennis.

## Reversibility

Simply stated, the principle of reversibility means you use it or lose it. When you stop exercising, the effects of your training will gradually be reduced. The rate at which it is reduced depends on your previous training and the length of your inactivity.

## Overload

The principle of overload states that for the body to make changes, as in getting stronger or more flexible, additional stress must be placed on the body. For example, if you perform biceps curls with 10-pound dumbbells and it is difficult, your body will eventually adapt (get stronger). To continue to increase your strength, you must add more stress, such as heavier dumbbells, additional sets, or more repetitions. This principle is used in all the components of fitness.

## Progression

Progression is the rate at which the overload is applied. A beginner should start slowly and gradually increase overload, which gives the body a chance to adapt and reduce the risk of injury or sore muscles. It also gives the connective tissue (ligaments and joints) and muscles time to adapt and prepare for higher-intensity workouts. The more unconditioned the exerciser, the slower the rate of progression.

In resistance training, more reps, weight, or sets are added. Cardiorespiratory progression should be made first by increasing time to at least 30 minutes before increasing intensity, such as the incline on a treadmill.

Understanding not only how to design a fitness program but how to implement these principles is important in helping you reach your fitness goals.

### SUCCESS CHECK

- ☒ Name four principles of training.
- ☒ How can the principles of training help you develop an exercise program?

# OVERVIEW OF FITNESS SUMMARY

Fitness is a life-long process, not something you accomplish and forget about. It includes several components, all equally important. Understanding the importance of these components, along with principles of training, will help you get on the right track to becoming fit. Remember, it's a journey that will help improve your quality of life, which will impact all that you do.

## Before Taking the Next Step

1. Locate an area in your home where you can perform your assessment.

2. Clear away any items that may get in your way.

3. Ask a friend or family member to assist you and set a date to complete your assessments.

# 2

# Testing and Evaluation

Testing and evaluation are an important part of fitness because they reveal information about your current health and fitness status. Without knowing where you are now, how will you know what direction to take? These measurements provide a baseline—a starting point that can help you establish goals and monitor progress as well as provide motivation.

The first part of testing is a health screening, including identifying risk factors for heart disease, blood pressure, pulse, body composition, and girth measurements. The second part is physical testing of balance, muscular strength and endurance, flexibility, and cardiorespiratory fitness. Finding out how you rate in each of these areas will help you design a fitness program that improves your weak areas and maintains your strong areas. At the end of this book is an assessment sheet for recording your health and fitness data.

## HEALTH SCREENING

The information in a health screening helps identify risk factors for heart disease and areas of risk for health and injury that may need the referral of a health professional before you start an exercise program. There are two simple tools to use in conducting health screening: a physical readiness questionnaire and an assessment of risk factors for heart disease.

The physical readiness questionnaire is a screening tool used to determine the safety or risk of anyone who is preparing to start an exercise program (see figure 2.1) Read each question carefully. According to the questionnaire, if you answered yes to one or more questions, consult a physician before taking a fitness test or starting an exercise program. If you answered no to all of the questions, you can be fairly sure that you can start a moderate exercise program without a physician's clearance.

## ASSESSING YOUR PHYSICAL READINESS

If you answer yes to any of the following questions, you should talk with your doctor *before* beginning a weight training program.

Yes     No

____    ____     Are you over age 55 (female) or 45 (male) and not accustomed to exercise?

____    ____     Do you have a history of heart disease?

____    ____     Has a doctor ever said your blood pressure was too high?

____    ____     Are you taking any prescription medications, such as those for heart problems or high blood pressure?

____    ____     Have you ever experienced chest pain, spells of severe dizziness, or fainting?

____    ____     Do you have a history of respiratory problems, such as asthma?

____    ____     Have you had surgery or had problems with your bones, muscles, tendons, or ligaments (especially in your back, shoulders, or knees) that might be aggravated by an exercise program?

____    ____     Is there a good physical or health reason not already mentioned here that you should not follow a weight training program?

**Figure 2.1** Physical readiness questionnaire.

Reprinted, by permission, from T.R. Baechle and R.W. Earle, 2014, *Fitness weight training*, 3rd ed. (Champaign, IL: Human Kinetics), 17.

# Risk Factors for Heart Disease

The online calculator at the American Heart Association's website is a comprehensive and easy-to-use tool. It estimates your risk of having a heart attack or dying from heart disease within the next 10 years. With the click of a mouse you will be asked questions about yourself such as age, height, weight, sex, and family history. You will also answer questions regarding your current health status, such as smoking, diabetes, and cholesterol. Keep in mind that the result of this screening for risk of heart disease is only an *estimate* and not a *prediction* of having a heart attack or heart disease in the near future. These results are not a medical report but a tool to help you decide if a physician's clearance is necessary before starting an exercise program. If your results indicate you are at risk, it's best to get a physician's clearance.

## SUCCESS CHECK

☒ Complete the questionnaire and the assessment of risk factors for heart disease. Log on to the American Heart Association's main and use the Attack Risk Calculator to see if you are at risk. Obtain a physician's clearance if needed.

# Blood Pressure

Blood pressure is the pressure exerted by circulating blood on the walls of blood vessels and is one of the principal vital signs. Systolic (top number) measures the pressure in the arteries when the heart contracts, and diastolic (bottom number) measures the pressure in the arteries when the heart muscle is resting between beats and refilling with blood. Many places offer blood pressure checks, including your doctor's office, pharmacies, workplace, health clubs, and local health events. You can also purchase your own automatic blood pressure cuff to use at home that is easy to use and has digital readouts.

Before checking your blood pressure, make sure you have an empty bladder and are comfortable and relaxed. Remove any tight-sleeved clothing, and rest 2 to 10 minutes. Your arm should be at heart level and feet flat on the floor. Place the cuff snugly an inch above the bend in your elbow and follow the directions on the blood pressure monitor. Compare your reading with table 2.1. If your systolic blood pressure reading is 140 or higher, or your diastolic blood pressure reading is 90 or higher (either number is high), consult your doctor. Proper exercise can lower blood pressure.

Table 2.1 Classification of Blood Pressure for Adults

| Systolic blood pressure | Diastolic blood pressure | Category |
|---|---|---|
| Normal | <120 | <80 |
| Prehypertension | 120-139 | 80-89 |
| Hypertension stage 1 | 140-159 | 90-99 |
| Hypertension stage 2 | >160 | >100 |

Source: U.S. Department of Health and Human Services, National Heart, Lung, and Blood Institute, *The seventh report of the Joint National Committee on Prevention, Detection, Evaluation, and Treatment of High Blood Pressure.* (Bethesda, MD: NIH Publication No. 03-5233, December 2003).

## SUCCESS CHECK

- ☒ Take your blood pressure reading. Make sure you sit and relax 10 minutes and keep your feet flat on the floor.
- ☒ Record your blood pressure on the assessment sheet. Is it within the normal range? If either number is high, consult your physician.

# Heart Rate

Your pulse is the rate at which your heart beats and is called your heart rate in exercise, which is the number of times your heart beats per minute (bpm). A normal resting heart rate can range from 40 to 100 bpm; the average is 60 to 80 bpm. The more cardiovascularly fit you are, the lower your resting heart rate due to the heart itself getting stronger and pumping blood more efficiently. Your heart does not have to work as hard!

Many factors can increase heart rate: stress, nicotine, illness, and hot weather. Increased resting heart rate in a physically fit person may indicate overtraining.

Performing a moderate cardio program five times per week for 30 minutes or an intense cardio program three times a week for 30 minutes can lower resting heart rate up to one beat per week.

According to the American Heart Association, the best time to calculate your resting heart rate is in the morning before you get out of bed. To take your pulse, do the following:

- Use your fingers when finding a pulse, because your thumb has a pulse of its own.
- Find the radial pulse on the inside of the wrist at the base of the thumb. You may also feel a pulse on your carotid arteries on either side of the neck.
- Count the beats for 10 seconds, starting with 0.
- Multiply by 6.
- Evaluate your resting heart rate using table 2.2.

Table 2.2   Normal Resting Heart Rates

| Adults (including seniors) | 60-100 beats per minute |
|---|---|
| Well-trained athletes | 40-60 beats per minute |

### SUCCESS CHECK

- ☒ Take your resting heart rate (pulse). Sit and relax for 10 minute before taking your pulse.
- ☒ Use your fingers, not your thumb.
- ☒ Press gently if you are using the neck site.
- ☒ Record your resting pulse on the assessment sheet. Is it within normal range?

## Body Composition

Your body is made up of fat mass and fat-free mass (muscle, bones, organs, and blood). Fat mass is essential for proper hormone production, function of the nervous system, protection of organs, and insulation. These normal body functions can be disrupted if body fat goes below the essential 5 percent for men and 8 percent for women. Without exercise, fat mass goes up 1 to 3 percent per decade after age 20 until age 60, when fat mass gradually declines.

### SKINFOLDS

Two people can be the same height and weight but look completely different because of their body compositions. To determine body composition, you must first find your percent or pounds of body fat. One way to determine your fat mass is by using skinfold measurements. A skinfold test measures the amount of fat directly under the skin, or subcutaneous fat, which is about 50 percent of your total body fat. Skin calipers are used to pinch the fat at various sites for men and women, and the sites can range from 3 to 9 depending on which skinfold test is administered. Results have a 3 to 5 percent chance of being too high or too low, but it is a good estimate. Because skill is needed in administering and evaluating this test, a professional should conduct the test to ensure accuracy.

## BIA

The bioelectric impedance assessment (BIA) is considered one of the most reliable and easy-to-use methods of determining body fat today. These devices ($25-$250) can be handheld or stepped on. The handheld device is most accurate for the upper body,

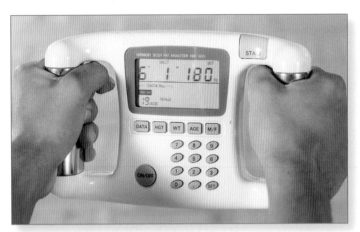

and the step-on device is most accurate for the lower body. See figure 2.2 for an example. The device sends a small electrical signal through the body that measures the resistance of the body's tissues. You will program in a few questions in regard to your age, weight, height, and sex. If you are using the handheld model, you will stand with your feet apart, extend your arms straight out, and hit the start button. In about seven seconds your percentage of body fat and pounds

**Figure 2.2**   Bioelectric impedance assessment device.

of fat will appear on the screen. For the step-on version, you must cover the electrodes with your bare feet and wait for the results to appear. Results have a 3 percent chance of being too high or too low, but it's a comparable assessment to the skinfold test. For the most accurate results, follow these guidelines:

- Do not eat or drink within 4 hours of the test.
- Do not exercise within 12 hours of the test.
- Urinate within 30 minutes of the test.
- Do not consume alcohol within 48 hours of the test.
- Do not take diuretics within 7 days of the test.

You should assess body composition once every six to eight weeks because the rate of fat loss is about 1 percent per month if you are unfit and untrained. Understand that additional weight may be lost, but the loss may be from water or muscle tissue.

## BMI

A third choice is an indirect measure, the body mass index (BMI), which uses height and weight to calculate body fat mass. It is widely used in schools and physicians' offices because the link between your BMI and fat is rather strong and the test is quick and easy to do, inexpensive, and practical.

Because it's an indirect measure, BMI does not take into consideration that although a man and woman may have the same BMI, men tend to carry less body fat than women. And the older population tends to carry more body fat than younger adults. In addition, those who have more muscle mass than the average person, such as athletes or soldiers, may show a high BMI (obesity) due to musculature, not fatness. For example, when basketball player Michael Jordan was at his best, his BMI was 29, which classified him as being overweight. However, his waist was under 30 inches! To determine your BMI, go to www.cdc.gov/healthyweight/assessing/bmi/adult_bmi/english_bmi_calculator/bmi_calculator.html or use figure 2.3.

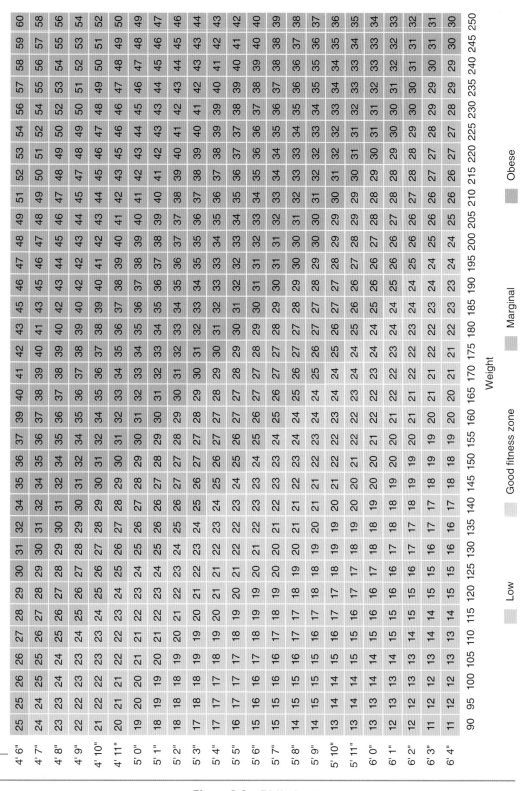

**Figure 2.3** BMI chart.

Reprinted, by permission, from C.B. Corbin and R. Lindsey, 2005, *Fitness for life*, 5th ed. (Champaign, IL: Human Kinetics), 81.

# Girth Measurements

Girth measurements are those that go around the body at specific anatomical sites, which include the chest, waist, hips, thigh, calf, and biceps. It's important to perform measurements periodically when starting an exercise program because it's common to lose girth instead of mass in the first six to eight weeks of an exercise program. The reason for this is twofold. First, your body is burning fat tissue (which takes up a lot of space) and building muscle tissue (which is much more compact). So it is possible to gain weight yet become smaller! Second, most people store body fat in the midsection, so losing girth around the middle means you are becoming leaner. This can be more motivating for you than the number on the scale if one of your fitness goals is to lose weight. You may notice your jeans getting baggy around your waistline yet your arms becoming lean and toned (more muscle). It's not uncommon for the scale to show a one- to two-pound increase after the first six to eight weeks when starting a program. Know not to get discouraged—anticipate it will happen!

On the other hand, if you want to increase muscle size, such as in your chest and biceps, girth measurements are an excellent way to monitor your progress. Knowing whether your muscles are growing may indicate you have reached a plateau or that your workout program needs to be changed.

Although there are specific tape measures that are spring-loaded, which makes this assessment easier to perform, it may be helpful to find someone who will measure you every four to six weeks using an inexpensive vinyl tape measure. Have the same person perform the assessment to ensure consistency.

Be consistent in using landmarks for each area. For the most accurate results, follow these guidelines and the instructions in table 2.3:

### Table 2.3  Body Measurement Guide

| Shoulders | Measure the circumference 2 inches below the bony tip of the shoulder. | 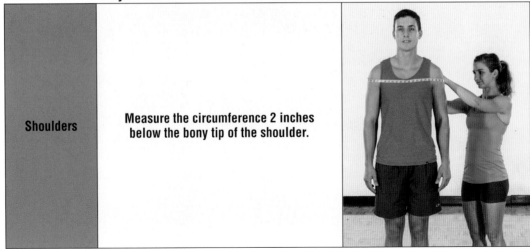 |
| --- | --- | --- |

| | | |
|---|---|---|
| **Chest: Men** | Measure the circumference at nipple level. | |
| **Chest: Women** | Measure the circumference of the upper chest (above breast). | |
| **Waist** | Measure the circumference of the smallest part of the waist. | |

*(continued)*

**Table 2.3** (continued)

| | | |
|---|---|---|
| Hips | Measure the circumference of the widest part of the glutes. | |
| Thigh | Measure the circumference midway between the hip bone and knee. | |
| Biceps | Measure the circumference midway between the shoulder and elbow. | |

- Wear tight-fitting clothing.
- Measure the right side of the body.
- Landmarks are marked for each measurement.
- Tape should be in contact with the body, not depressing the skin.
- Use a mirror to ensure the tape is level.

## SUCCESS CHECK

- ☒ Use a Myotape or ask someone to take your measurements.
- ☒ Record your measurements on the assessment sheet.

# Posture

Posture refers to the body's alignment and positioning in regard to gravity. Whether you are standing, walking, playing, sleeping, or working, gravity imposes a force on the joints, connective tissue, and muscles that affects health. Poor posture affects not only physical movement and its efficiency but also digestion, elimination, and breathing. Poor posture results from a combination of several factors:

- Occupational stress
- Muscle imbalances (muscles that are either too weak or not flexible)
- Excessive weight
- Poor mattress
- Injuries, falls, and accidents
- Poorly designed work space
- Improper footwear and foot problems

Good posture alleviates stress on joints, helps muscles function properly, prevents back pain, reduces fatigue, and aids in a good appearance. Therefore, proper posture is an extremely important factor in your assessment. Without good posture, you cannot be physically fit or function efficiently. Determining muscle imbalances (what needs to be stretched and what needs to be strengthened) is vital in designing a fitness program.

The easiest posture analysis is a visual assessment that can indicate any problem areas you may have. You may also choose the expertise of your local chiropractor who can make assessments and recommendations. To evaluate your posture, face a full-length mirror wearing tight clothes. Closing your eyes, take a few deep breaths and relax into your normal postural stance. It may help to have a family member or friend with you to snap a picture from the front and side angles. Use table 2.4 to assess your posture.

### Table 2.4 Guidelines for Evaluating Posture

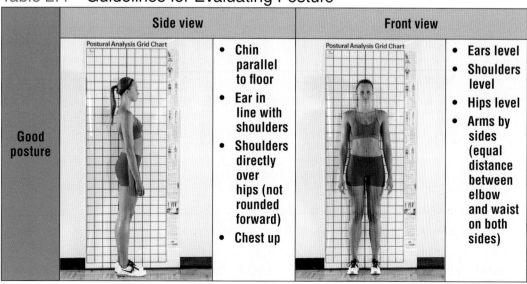

| | Side view | | Front view | |
|---|---|---|---|---|
| Good posture | Postural Analysis Grid Chart | • Chin parallel to floor<br>• Ear in line with shoulders<br>• Shoulders directly over hips (not rounded forward)<br>• Chest up | Postural Analysis Grid Chart | • Ears level<br>• Shoulders level<br>• Hips level<br>• Arms by sides (equal distance between elbow and waist on both sides) |

*(continued)*

**Table 2.4** *(continued)*

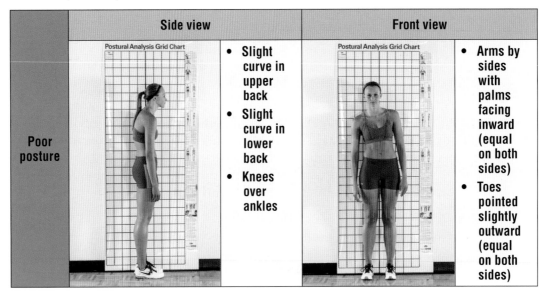

| | Side view | Front view |
|---|---|---|
| **Poor posture** | • Slight curve in upper back<br>• Slight curve in lower back<br>• Knees over ankles | • Arms by sides with palms facing inward (equal on both sides)<br>• Toes pointed slightly outward (equal on both sides) |

## SUCCESS CHECK

- ☒ Evaluate your posture. How do these assessments help you evaluate your fitness?
- ☒ Record the results on the assessment sheet.

# PHYSICAL TESTING

Physical testing will best indicate your fitness level. Specific areas of your body and muscles perform specific functions that may need to be strengthened or stretched, depending on your daily activities. Physical testing includes various levels of balance tests, a push-up test for upper-body strength, a squat test for lower-body strength, and a curl-up test for core strength.

## Balance

Proprioception (balance) is the body's ability to understand and use information about body position in space. It allows you to control your limbs without looking at them. Signals from the soles of your feet, the relation of your inner ear to gravity, and what you see prompt the body to activate or deactivate muscles in order to maintain your preferred position. It does this every time you stand, go down steps, lift weights, get dressed, pick up a child, or stand on tiptoe. Increasing your ability to balance will improve coordination and posture (as well as athletic skill) and will result in increased stability and fewer injuries. The following figures show three balance tests to try.

## ONE-LEG BALANCE TEST

Ask a friend or family member to time you. Adults should be able to balance 30 seconds:

1. Stand on a hard surface as demonstrated in figure 2.4.
2. Raise one foot off the floor, bending the knee at a 90-degree angle.
3. Close your eyes and start the timer. If you have difficulty performing this test, you can keep your eyes open.
4. Stop timing if eyes open, the foot lowers, or you begin teetering.
5. Repeat three times and calculate the average.

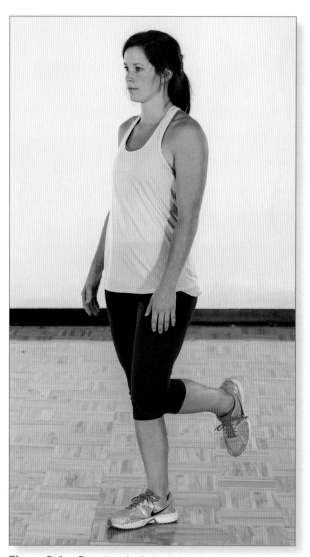

**Figure 2.4**   One-leg balance test.

## RHOMBERG AND SHARPENED RHOMBERG BALANCE TESTS

There are two versions of this test shown in figures 2.5*a* and 2.5*b*, depending on your ability. If the body sways on either test, balance can be improved.

1. Stand with feet together and arms crossed over the upper chest.
2. Close eyes and start the timer.
3. Observe for one full minute.
4. Stand with feet heel to toe with arms crossed over the upper chest.
5. Close eyes and start the timer.
6. Observe for one full minute.

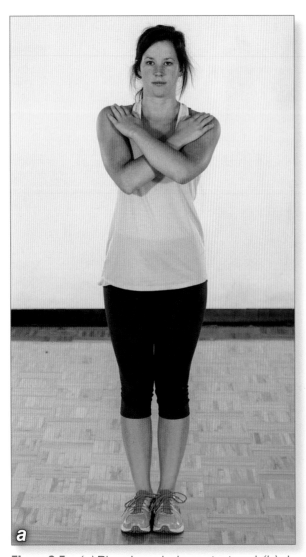 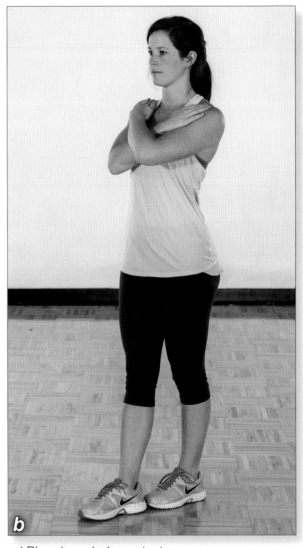

**Figure 2.5** *(a)* Rhomberg balance test and *(b)* sharpened Rhomberg balance test.

## STORK STAND TEST

This is a more advanced option that tests not only your balance but also your balance endurance. Take the best out of three trials. Stop timing if your hands come off your hips, your foot comes off your leg, your support foot moves, or your heel touches the floor. See figure 2.6 for a demonstration.

1. Stand barefoot on a hard surface.
2. Place hands on hips.
3. Stand on one leg, making contact anywhere below the knee with the other leg.
4. Raise the heel of the support leg off the floor and start timing.
5. Repeat on other leg.
6. Take the best out of three tries for each leg.
7. Try to hold this position for 10 seconds.

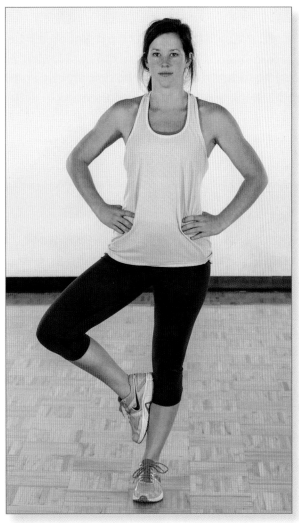

**Figure 2.6** Stork stand test.

## SUCCESS CHECK

☒ Perform the balance assessments for yourself and record the results on the assessment sheet. What conclusions can you draw based on the results?

## Upper-Body Strength and Endurance

A good indication of overall fitness is strength and endurance in the muscles of the upper body, especially the chest, shoulders, triceps, and core. Strength and endurance in the upper body are important for anyone performing daily activities such as carrying groceries, picking up a book bag, or carrying laundry baskets without difficulty and without risk of injury. The majority of lifetime and competitive sports also depend on strong upper-body muscular strength and endurance to help support the spine and maintain balance.

Each muscle in the upper body has a role that affects everyday movement. Many times overuse of a muscle in a sport, activity, or job can cause muscle imbalance—stronger muscles in the front than back, or stronger muscles on the left side than the right side of the body. The push-up test, shown in figures 2.7 and 2.8 and the corresponding figures (2.9*a* and 2.9*b*), is a common fitness test that evaluates upper-body strength and endurance.

### PUSH-UP TEST

- Start in the down position with front nearly flat on the floor.
- Men must perform regular (on toes) push-ups; women may perform modified (on knees) push-ups or perform the one-minute standard push-up test.
- Push up until arms are fully extended, then lower within 4 inches of the floor.
- Do as many as you can; this test is not timed.

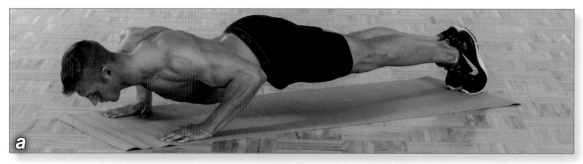

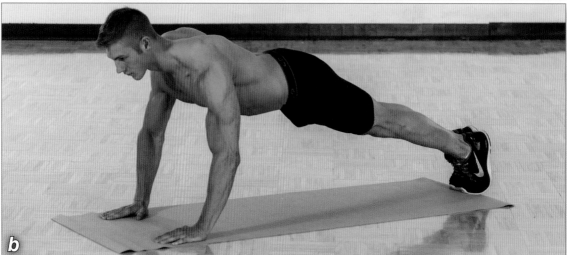

**Figure 2.7**   Proper standard push-up form.

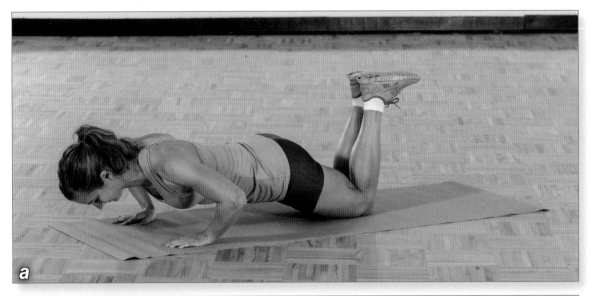

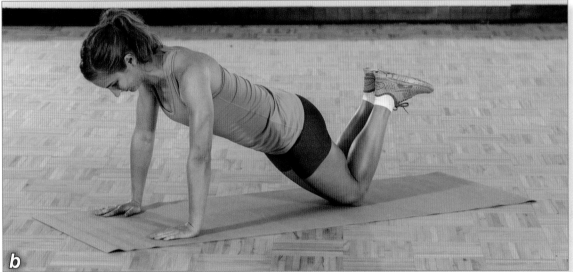

**Figure 2.8** Proper modified push-up form.

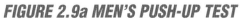

## FIGURE 2.9a MEN'S PUSH-UP TEST

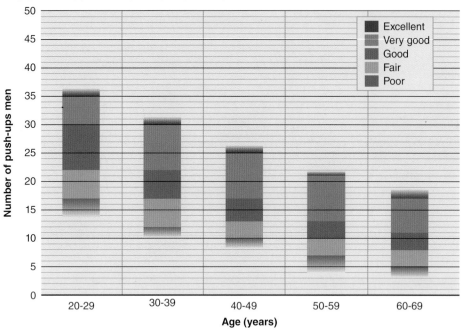

Adapted from Canadian Society of Exercise Physiology, 2003, *The Canadian physical activity, fitness & lifestyle approach: CSEP-Health & Fitness Program's health-related appraisal & counselling strategy* (Ottawa, ON: CSEP), 7-47.

## FIGURE 2.9b WOMEN'S PUSH-UP TEST

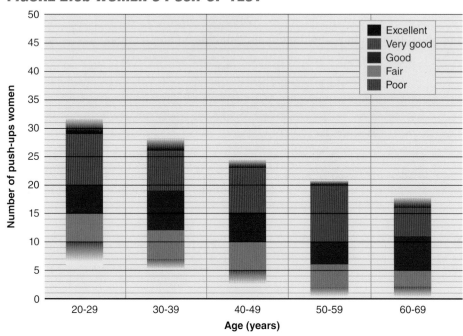

Adapted from Canadian Society of Exercise Physiology, 2003, *The Canadian physical activity, fitness & lifestyle approach: CSEP-Health & Fitness Program's health-related appraisal & counselling strategy* (Ottawa, ON: CSEP), 7-48.

   ☒  Perform the push-up test.

   ☒  Record your score on the assessment sheet.

# Abdominal Endurance

The curl-up test as shown in figures 2.10, 2.11*a*, and 2.11*b* measures abdominal strength and endurance. It is a safer and more reliable indicator of abdominal strength than a full sit-up because it does not involve the powerful hip flexor muscles. Strong abdominals not only help support the spine and provide with good posture, but they also aid in balance and functional movement. Any movement from the arms or legs either originates or travels through the core.

## CURL-UP TEST

- Place two strips of tape 3.5 inches (almost 9 cm) apart on the floor or use the edge of a mat.
- Lie on your back with your fingertips touching the first strip of tape, or 3.5 inches from the edge of the mat, shoulders relaxed.
- Bend knees; do not have anyone hold your feet.
- Curl up until your fingertips touch the second strip of tape, or the end of the mat, and down until your shoulders touch the floor, keeping your hands in contact with the floor at all times.
- Do as many as you can for 1 minute.

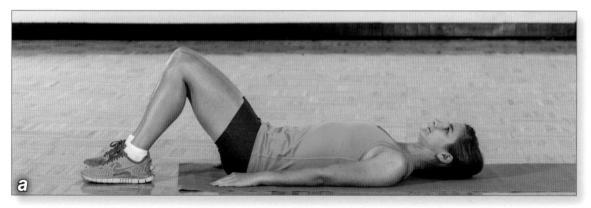

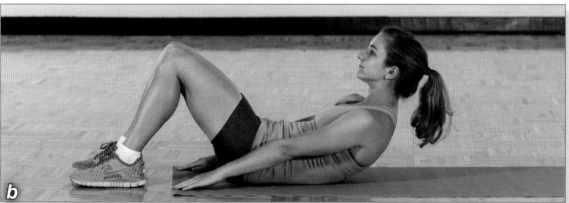

**Figure 2.10**  Proper curl-up form.

### FIGURE 2.11a MEN'S CURL-UP TEST

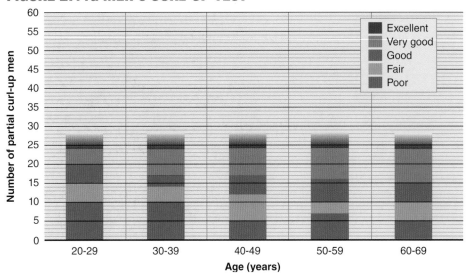

Adapted from Canadian Society of Exercise Physiology, 2003, *The Canadian physical activity, fitness & lifestyle approach: CSEP-Health & Fitness Program's health-related appraisal & counselling strategy* (Ottawa, ON: CSEP), 7-47.

### FIGURE 2.11b WOMEN'S CURL-UP TEST

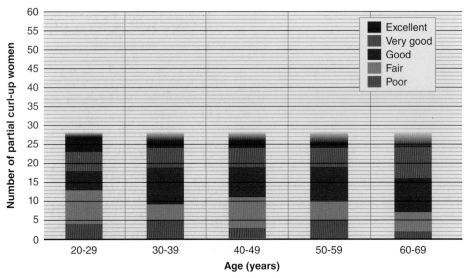

Adapted from Canadian Society of Exercise Physiology, 2003, *The Canadian physical activity, fitness & lifestyle approach: CSEP-Health & Fitness Program's health-related appraisal & counselling strategy* (Ottawa, ON: CSEP), 7-48.

## SUCCESS CHECK

- ☒ Perform the curl-up test and record your score.
- ☒ Record your score on the assessment sheet.

# Lower-Body Strength and Endurance

Your base of support as you run, walk, climb stairs, or sit in a chair is the lower body, where the largest muscles of the body are located. Lower-body strength and endurance are important for stamina, joint stabilization, balance, and mobility, which can make daily activities easier as well as help prevent overuse injuries. Lower-body strength and endurance are extremely important for those who participate in lifetime or competitive sport activities.

Many people have the misconception that they don't need to train the lower body if they perform a great deal of cardiorespiratory exercise! These are the largest muscles in the body, and they support half of you in addition to increasing bone strength. So of course you need to keep them strong!

## *WALL SIT*

- Stand with your back flat against the wall, feet 12 inches (30 cm) from the wall.
- Lower your body until thighs are parallel to the floor, making a right angle as demonstrated in figure 2.12.
- Start the timer and use figures 2.13*a* and 2.13*b* as a reference.

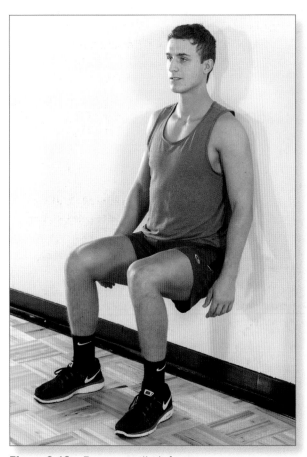

**Figure 2.12**   Proper wall sit form.

### FIGURE 2.13a MEN'S WALL SIT TEST

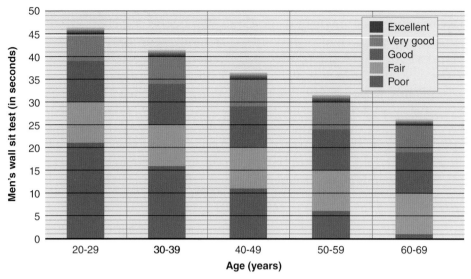

Adapted from information available at www.thefitmap.co.uk/exercise/tests/strength/lower/wall.htm [accessed October20, 2014].

### FIGURE 2.13b WOMEN'S WALL SIT TEST

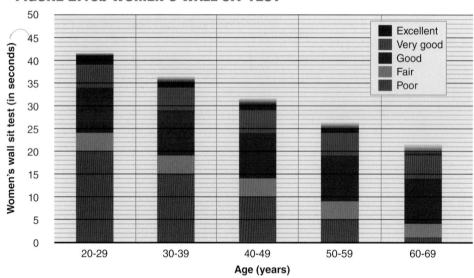

Adapted from information available at www.thefitmap.co.uk/exercise/tests/strength/lower/wall.htm [accessed October20, 2014].

### SUCCESS CHECK

- ☒ Perform the wall sit test.
- ☒ Record your score on the assessment sheet.

# Flexibility

Flexibility is the range of motion around a joint. Without range of motion, muscles cannot function properly, which may affect daily activities or sport performance. Loss of flexibility can also lead to pain or balance disorders. Factors that affect flexibility include sex, age, genetics, joint structure, muscle imbalance, injuries, fat, and activity level.

Because flexibility deteriorates with age, it's important to maintain the flexibility you now have. Loss of flexibility brings loss of mobility, which in turn brings loss of stability. The results are greater risk of falls and loss of independence. The pass–fail flexibility tests in table 2.5 will help you determine the joint areas that are normal and those that are tight and need improvement. Warm up a few minutes before performing, and don't stretch to the point of pain.

Table 2.5   Flexibility Guidelines

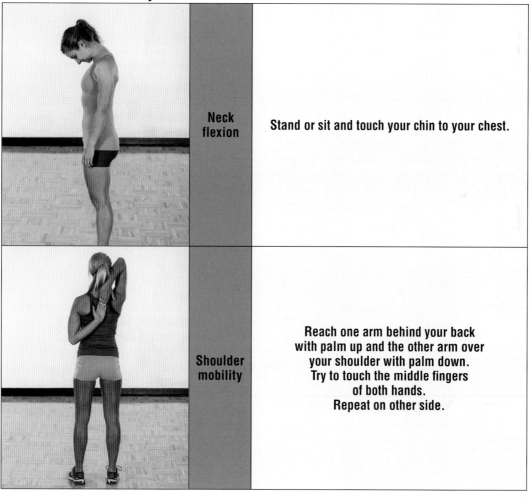

| | Neck flexion | Stand or sit and touch your chin to your chest. |
| | Shoulder mobility | Reach one arm behind your back with palm up and the other arm over your shoulder with palm down. Try to touch the middle fingers of both hands. Repeat on other side. |

(continued)

**Table 2.5** *(continued)*

| | Shoulder flexion | Stand and raise straight arm slowly to the front until it reaches overhead. Repeat on other side. |
| --- | --- | --- |
| | Shoulder abduction | Stand and raise straight arm to the side until it reaches overhead. Repeat on other side. |
| | Trunk rotation | Sit with feet flat and ball or block between knees. Cross arms on chest. Rotate slowly to right to 45°. Repeat to left. |
| | Low back | Sit on the floor with legs straight. Slowly lean forward and touch your toes. |

| | | |
|---|---|---|
| | Ham-string | Lie on back with arms by sides. Keeping both legs straight, slowly lift one leg up to 90 degrees. |
| | Hip flexor | Lie on your back with legs straight. Slowly bring one knee to the chest. Opposite leg should stay flat against the floor. Repeat on other side. |
| | Calf | Sit with legs straight and feet together, toes pointing up. Slowly flex one foot 30 degrees. Repeat on other side. |
| | Quad | Lie on your front with your forehead resting on your hand. Touch the heel to the glute. Repeat on other side. |

## SUCCESS CHECK

- ☒ Perform the pass–fail flexibility tests.
- ☒ Record your results on the assessment sheet.

# Cardiorespiratory Fitness

The heart is the most important muscle in the body, so cardiorespiratory fitness (strong heart and lungs) is considered the most important component of physical fitness. Your heart is responsible for distributing oxygen to every working muscle. This in turn has a direct impact on everyday movements as well as sport performance.

Maximal cardio tests are performed in a clinical setting with a team of people. You can easily perform a submaximal cardiorespiratory test that will indicate how your cardiorespiratory fitness compares to the norms. The test listed here will help you identify your cardiorespiratory fitness using time as a measurement.

Either test can be completed on a treadmill or outdoors on a track. As another option, many of today's cardio machines have fitness tests built into the machines.

## 1-MILE WALK TEST

This test measures how quickly you can walk a mile—you are looking at *time*. You will need (ideally) a track, but you can also use a treadmill and a stopwatch. You could even take the test in your neighborhood, provided you choose a completely flat area with no inclines. You can mark out a one-mile route with a car odometer or use a tool like the USATF's course calculator. This would also be a good time to measure your heart rate after the test is completed.

- Warm up by walking for 5 minutes.
- Start your stopwatch and walk 1 mile as fast as you can, but don't run.
- At the end of 1 mile, stop and record the time. Use table 2.6 as a reference.

Table 2.6  Norms for the 1-Mile Walk Test

| Rating | Age 18-30 | | Age 31-69 | |
|---|---|---|---|---|
| | Men | Women | Men | Women |
| Excellent | <11:08 | <11:45 | <10:12 | <11:40 |
| Good | 11:42-11:09 | 12:49-11:46 | 10:13-11:42 | 11:41-13:08 |
| High average | 12:38-11:41 | 13:15-12:50 | 11:43-13:13 | 13:09-14:36 |
| Low average | 13:38-12:37 | 14:12-13:16 | 13:14-14:44 | 14:37-16:04 |
| Fair | 14:37-13:37 | 15:03-14:13 | 14:45-16:23 | 16:05-17:31 |
| Poor | >14:38 | >15:04 | >16:24 | >17:32 |

Adapted, by permission, from J.R. Morrow, A.W. Jackson, J.G. Disch, and D.P. Mood, 2005, *Measurement and evaluation in human performance, 3rd ed.* (Champaign, IL: Human Kinetics), 235.

## SUCCESS CHECK

- [x] Perform the 1-mile walk test.
- [x] Record the results on the assessment sheet.

# TESTING AND EVALUATION SUMMARY

Now that you have completed your health screening and fitness assessment, you should know the areas that need work and the areas that you need to maintain. Use this information as you read the next step on setting goals. Although you may have other goals you would like to accomplish, such as losing weight or running a 5K, don't forget to include any area in which you scored low.

If your shoulders were tight, your balance was off, or your upper body was weak, use the next step to write goals so that these areas can be improved. If you are a beginning exerciser, it is helpful to complete a reassessment in the areas in which you scored poorly about every four to six weeks. Remember that it took time to get out of shape, and it will take time to get back into shape.

## Before Taking the Next Step

1. Did you complete the physical readiness questionnaire or the heart disease risk factor assessment?

2. Did you obtain a physician's clearance, if necessary?

3. Did you record your blood pressure and resting heart rate?

4. Did you record your body composition and measurements?

5. Did you complete the posture and balance tests?

6. Have you performed and recorded the muscular strength and endurance tests for upper body, lower body, and abdominals? Did you complete all the flexibility tests and record the results?

7. Did you choose a cardio test and record the result?

# 3

# Goals

Setting goals is one of the most overlooked but most important aspects of a successful fitness plan. Goals not only help identify what you want to accomplish but how to go about accomplishing the goals. In this step you will learn about SMART goals and how to set both short- and long-term goals that will lead you through your journey to becoming fit. You will also learn the difference between result-oriented goals and behavior-oriented goals and which ones are the best for you. More important, you will understand the time frame involved in reaching your goals safely through current industry standards.

## SMART GOALS

SMART is an acronym that helps clarify your fitness goals. Having a general goal such as wanting to lose weight or wanting to be fit makes it difficult to devise a plan of action to accomplish those goals or document progress. A SMART goal is a map that leads you to your destination.

### Start With Specifics

The S in SMART stands for *specific*. Every goal should be clearly defined. Instead of making a general statement as a goal, such as "I want to lose weight," you must be more specific. You must answer the *who*, *what*, and *where* to determine how you are going to achieve weight loss. There are several ways to lose weight, including eliminating sweets, performing cardiorespiratory exercises, strength training, and reducing calories. "I want to lose 10 pounds by doing an hour of cardiorespiratory exercise and strength training" is a specific goal. Another specific goal is "I want to lose 10 pounds by walking an hour four times a week and eliminating sweets."

Another example is stating a general goal of becoming more fit. There are many ways to be more fit, such as stopping smoking, increasing your intake of fruits and vegetables, walking, and participating in yoga classes. A more specific goal is to be more fit by walking 30 minutes five times per week and eating five fruits and vegetables daily for the next three months. Having specific goals not only will help you be more focused but will also help you design a fitness program specifically for you depending on your daily schedule and exercise preferences.

## Measure Your Progress

The M in SMART stands for *measureable*. You must be able to measure the goals you set. If your goal is to lose 10 pounds, you can measure your weight by stepping on a scale. If your goal is to exercise three times per week for one hour for three months, you can measure that by marking off the days of the week and documenting the time you exercised. If your goal is to lose body fat, you can measure it by skinfold calipers or a bioelectrical analysis machine.

Ask yourself how you will track your progress. Recording your progress not only will help you stay on track but will also help keep you motivated. You will feel more committed, stronger, and well organized by taking charge of documenting your achievements, which can lead to positive thoughts about yourself and inspire you to reach your goal and stay focused.

There are several ways to track your progress. You can simply use a notebook to jot down your weight, percentage of fat, BMI, blood pressure, and any other information you want to track every week or month. Free websites also will track fitness data, such as livestrong.com and myfitnesspal.com. Those with iPhones can use apps such as the Argus app or Fitbit app. Also available for those who don't own an iPhone are tracking devices such as the Fitbit Tracker or Nike+ Sport band.

## Keep Your Perspective

The A in SMART stands for *attainable*. This is where many people become dropouts. Although you may want to set the bar high, you will be setting yourself up for failure if you are not in a place to achieve it. A goal of losing 10 pounds in a weekend is not attainable; a goal of losing 1 to 2 pounds per week is attainable. You may state that you are going to work out every day only to find that life gets in the way and you have missed three days in a row. A goal of working out for three hours for someone who is currently a couch potato may not be attainable, and it will increase the risk of injury. Goals must fit into your time schedule, fitness level, and exercise preference. Stating you will exercise 30 to 60 minutes three times a week by walking on the treadmill and performing a circuit of weight training is an attainable goal. It's important to know your own personal habits, such as what time of the day is best to exercise or how late you schedule your last meal, so that you are able to gauge how much of a change is reasonable in obtaining a fitness goal. For example, if you are not a morning person, don't schedule a 6:00 a.m. workout. If you work late and come home famished, don't choose a nutrition goal of not eating after 7:00 p.m.

## Focus Your Intentions

The R in SMART stands for *relevant*. Your goals need to be related to your abilities, interests, and needs. Goals should be something you want to work toward; they should not set you up for failure. If you abhor running, don't make your goal training for a 5K race. If you do not like Spinning classes do not sign up for a month of Spinning classes or purchase an exercise bike for your home. Another example is instead of saying you will never eat another dessert, say that you will limit your desserts to twice a week.

## Keep Track of Time

The T in SMART stands for *time bound*. It is critical to set a time limit in order to accomplish your goals. Are you a procrastinator? Set a specific time for you to accomplish the goal so that you stay motivated, which will entice you to get moving. How can you make a change without choosing a deadline for meeting your goals? Therefore, losing 10 pounds in the next 8 weeks or exercising 30 to 60 minutes three times a week for the next month are time-bound goals.

One reason many people stop exercising after they make their New Year's resolutions is that exercise just becomes an activity like an endless chore with no direction. Having a concrete list of achievable goals can go a long way in helping you stick to your resolutions.

# LONG- AND SHORT-TERM GOALS

When setting goals, you need both long-term and short-term goals. You want to look at the big picture, but you also want to look at the baby steps (short-term goals) that will take you to that result (long-term goal). Short-term goals can be daily, weekly, or monthly goals. And depending on your current health and fitness status, long-term goals can last one month or up to a year.

Although you may have many goals you want to reach, it is important to focus on a few at a time. Choosing one long-term goal and two or three short-term goals will give you a better chance at accomplishment. Once you complete them, you can set new goals. Remember that short-term goals are used as steps in changing your behavior, or reaching your long-term goal.

Later in this step, you will learn the answer to a common question everyone asks: "How long until I see results?" We discuss industry standards in safely reaching your fitness goals and how quickly you can reach them. Once you complete the writing of your goals, make sure they meet industry standards for both expectations and safety. You may have to adjust your goals as you read through this information.

The SMART Goals Sample Worksheet in table 3.1*a* offers ideas on recording your specific fitness goals. Use the SMART acronym to write one long-term goal and three short-term goals. Make your goals SMART and you will be more likely to achieve them!

Table 3.1*b* is a sample worksheet to use for your own goals. After you list your goals and a timeline for achieving them, you need to identify the barriers and solutions to that will help you reach your goal. Use table 3.2*a* as an example and 3.2*b* to identify your own barriers and solutions.

Table 3.1*a*   SMART Goal Sample Worksheet

| Long-term goal | Plan (name 3 key actions needed to achieve this goal) | Start and end dates |
|---|---|---|
| I will lose 25 pounds in the next 6 months. | 1. Walk 30 minutes 3 days a week. 2. Perform a circuit of strength training twice a week. 3. Schedule my workout days in my planner. | Start: Jan 1 End: June 1 |

| Short-term goals | Plan (name 3 key actions needed to achieve this goal) | Start and end dates |
|---|---|---|
| Consume 5 fruits and vegetables daily. | 1. Purchase a variety of fruits and vegetables at the supermarket.<br>2. Wash and prep all fruits and vegetables.<br>3. Prepare individual servings for convenience. | Start: Jan 1<br>End: Jan 7 |
| Join a yoga class. | 1. Search the area for yoga classes and schedules.<br>2. Register and pay for yoga class.<br>3. Buy yoga mat and water bottle. | Start: Feb 9<br>End: Mar 16 |
| Design a strength training program for the first 3 weeks of training. | 1. Choose 1 exercise per muscle group.<br>2. Perform 1 set of 12 to 15 repetitions.<br>3. Increase weight when I can do 15 reps with proper form and technique. | Start: Jan 2<br>End: Jan 23 |

## Table 3.1b   My SMART goals

| Long-term goal | Plan (name 3 key actions needed to achieve this goal) | Start and end dates |
|---|---|---|
|  | 1. |  |
|  | 2. |  |
|  | 3. |  |

**Reward** when goal is reached:

| Short-term goals | Plan (name 3 key actions needed to achieve this goal) | Start and end dates |
|---|---|---|
| 1. | 1. |  |
| 2. | 2. |  |
| 3. | 3. |  |

**Reward** when goal is reached:

From N.L. Naternicola, 2015, *Fitness: Steps to success* (Champaign, IL: Human Kinetics).

Table 3.2*a*  Barriers to Goals and Their Solutions

| Barrier | Solution |
|---|---|
| 1.  Yoga class is too expensive | 1.  Purchase or rent yoga DVD. |
| 2.  I'm not sure what to do when eating out with friends. | 1.  Eat a healthy snack beforehand.<br>2.  Drink lemon water while waiting for food. |
| 3.  I'm not sure what exercises to do for upper body. | 1.  Write down upper-body muscle groups.<br>2.  Search online for exercises specific to each muscle. |

Table 3.2*b*  Barriers to My Goals and Their Solutions

| Barrier | Solution |
|---|---|
| 1. | 1. |
| 2. | 2. |
| 3. | 3. |

From N.L. Naternicola, 2015, *Fitness: Steps to success* (Champaign, IL: Human Kinetics).

## SUCCESS CHECK

- ☒ Write one long-term goal using the SMART acronym.
- ☒ Write three short-term goals using the SMART acronym.

# RESULT-ORIENTED GOALS AND BEHAVIOR-ORIENTED GOALS

Short- and long-term goals can either be result-oriented or behavior-oriented goals. Deciding which type of goal is appropriate depends not only on what you want to accomplish but also on knowing your past attempts and what might work best for you. It also depends on your fitness level.

A result-oriented goal is one that focuses on results, such as losing 10 pounds, lowering blood pressure, or running a race in a certain time. These goals are based solely on the outcome, and most people focus on these types of goals.

A behavior-oriented goal is one that focuses on changing a behavior. These goals focus on behavior, such as exercising one hour three times a week for the next month. This goal is specific, measureable, attainable, relevant, and time bound. But it is based on the behavior, not results. Of course, a bonus is that you would also lose weight in the process, but losing weight is not mentioned; only the behavior, or process, of losing weight is mentioned.

You need to decide what type of goal would be best for you. Setting goals is very personal, and goals should be based on what *you* want to accomplish. Usually behavior goals work best if you are currently inactive or sedentary, because they help you include exercise as part of a weekly routine. After time, exercise will become part of your life without having to write it as a goal.

An example of a long-term behavior goal is exercising an hour a day five times a week for the next year. A short-term behavior goal is exercising 15 minutes three times a week for the next three weeks. The time can be increased by five minutes every three weeks, and once you can exercise for an hour the days can be increased from three times a week to four times a week, then five times a week. Increasing your exercise to five times a week should happen gradually over several months to help reduce the risk of injury as well as fit in your schedule.

### SUCCESS CHECK

- ☒ Write one result-oriented goal.
- ☒ Write one behavior-oriented goal.

# HOW SOON CAN I SEE RESULTS?

The age-old question is "How long is this going to take?" In other words, how fast can you see results? Regardless of what you see on television or read in magazines, losing weight and becoming fit take time. It takes time to get out of shape, and it takes time to get back into shape. There is no magic pill or specific way to exercise that will whip you into shape more quickly. We discuss how fast certain components of exercise can be achieved, and your goals should reflect the appropriate time that it will take to reach certain aspects of your fitness program. It does not happen overnight regardless of what infomercial you see on the television.

Remember that getting fit and staying fit are a lifestyle. It is a journey and not a destination, which means periodically you must evaluate your goals. Once you reach your goals, you need to set new ones. Now that you have completed the health screening and physical fitness testing in step 2, you can determine your goals based on the initial data and decide whether you need to improve in a specific area or maintain the habits you have.

## Cardiorespiratory Fitness

Your resting heart rate is a good indicator of your cardiorespiratory fitness. The lower your resting heart rate, the more fit you are because your heart does not have to work so hard in pumping blood throughout your body. Beginners and those who are unfit who start performing 30 minutes of cardiorespiratory workouts a minimum of three times a week at the correct intensity level can lower their resting heart rate up to one beat per week. Within 10 weeks it is possible to lower resting heart rate by 10! Your heart will be pumping the same amount of blood to the working muscles with fewer beats because you are strengthening the heart muscle. You will send oxygen to your  working muscles more quickly, which will enhance your performance in anything you do. Besides having more energy and sleeping better, you will also begin to feel better.

Following are sample cardiorespiratory goals based on different people and outcomes:

- **Student**: I will go to the student rec center after my classes on Monday, Wednesday, and Friday and do 15 minutes on a cardio machine with my heart rate between 145 and 155 and increase my time by 5 minutes every week until I can do 30 minutes.
- **Soccer mom**: This fall, 5 days a week while my son is practicing, I will walk or run around the soccer field for 30 minutes until I can complete 30 minutes of running.

## Muscular Strength and Endurance

Seeing results for muscular strength and endurance is more complicated because it depends on several factors as well as muscle fiber type and workout design. These factors include nutrition, body type, age, and workout design. It also depends on what your goal is for your muscles. Do you want to increase muscle mass? Do you want to increase muscular endurance? Do you want to increase muscular strength? We discuss each of these and give you an idea to determine how fast you can reach these goals. It is also important to note that muscles can be built at any age!

### INCREASING MUSCLE MASS

Muscle mass depends on the number and type of muscle fibers (cells) you were born with. The two specific types of muscle fibers are slow-twitch (type I) and fast-twitch (type II). Fast-twitch muscle fibers are further categorized into type IIa and type IIb muscle fibers. The more type IIb muscle fibers you have, the more likely you are to gain muscle mass. Type IIb muscle fibers are used for power, speed, and size. Slow-twitch muscle fibers are used for endurance activities such as walking, running, and aerobics. These fibers are also used for repeated movements such as push-ups and crunches. Fast-twitch muscle fibers are used for short, fast, powerful movement such as sprinting and jumping.

Male beginners who lift heavy weights with low repetitions two or three times a week typically gain one pound of muscle per month for about six months; women see slower progress because they have smaller muscles. Usually both male and female beginners can see a gain of two to four pounds of muscle the first three months of lifting weights. If your goal is to lose weight, it is important to take into consideration lean muscle that you will be acquiring. Remember that muscle burns calories 24/7, so the more muscle you have, the more calories you burn.

### INCREASING MUSCULAR ENDURANCE

Again, muscular endurance depends on how many slow-twitch type I muscle fibers you have. These fibers are known for using oxygen better, which provides more fuel when performing exercise over a long period, such as running, biking, or swimming as summarized in table 3.3. These fibers are resistant to fatigue and respond to exercises that use low weight and high repetitions. Depending on your current fitness status, building muscular endurance can take anywhere from six weeks to more than three months. You should really begin to have more energy and feel better within the first four weeks.

One more factor to think about when talking about muscle is that type IIa muscle fibers are considered a combination of slow- and fast-twitch fibers because they can

Table 3.3   Types of Muscle Fibers

| Slow-twitch muscle fibers | Fast-twitch muscle fibers |
|---|---|
| Use oxygen more efficiently (aerobic)<br>Fire slowly<br>Red in color<br>Fatigue resistant | Anaerobic<br>Fire quickly<br>White in color<br>Fatigue quickly |
| **Good for** | **Good for** |
| Long energy needs such as running and biking | Short bursts of energy such as sprinting |

take on the characteristics of either fast- or slow-twitch muscle fibers depending on your workout design. If you are performing weight training exercises with heavy weight and low repetitions, these muscle fibers take on type IIb characteristics. However, if you are performing exercises with low weight and high repetitions, they will take on the characteristics of slow-twitch muscle fibers. That is why it is important to have an exercise program suitable for your goals.

It is also important to understand that muscle fibers cannot be changed into type I or type II fibers. Genetics determine which type and the amount of muscle fibers your body has.

## INCREASING MUSCULAR STRENGTH

Acquiring muscular strength happens much sooner than acquiring mass or muscular endurance. Within three weeks you may be stronger; however, it is important to understand that your neurological system will be recruiting muscle fibers that have not been used during the first three weeks of weight training. This process is called motor learning because your muscles respond to the challenging workload in your exercise program.

Following are examples of muscular strength and endurance goals:

- **Beginner**: I will increase muscular endurance by completing one set of 12 to 15 repetitions doing a circuit of weight machine exercises three times a week for four weeks.

- **Advanced**: I will increase my upper-body strength by completing 3 sets of 12 repetitions doing exercises for my chest, back, shoulders, and arms three times a week for six weeks.

## Fat Loss

There is a difference between weight loss and fat loss. The average person can safely lose one to two pounds (0.5-1 kg) of fat per week, which requires a deficit of 3,500 calories for each pound of body fat lost. Although there may be more weight lost according to the scale, the additional weight may be water or muscle. Without proper nutrition and exercise, your body can end up burning the muscle tissue you so desperately want to gain.

Remember that it is normal for a beginning exerciser to gain a few pounds at first when building lean mass, so it is equally important to track your lean body mass and body fat to make sure you are losing fat tissue, not lean body tissue. Your body consists of two categories of mass: fat mass and fat-free mass. Fat mass is purely fat (adipose). Fat-free mass (also known as lean mass) includes muscles, bones, organs, and blood. Because your bones, organs, and blood usually don't change after puberty, an increase or decrease in fat-free mass is a good indicator of gaining or losing muscle. You do not want to lose hard-earned calorie-burning muscle tissue!

Overall, you can safely lose 1 to 2 percent of fat per month. This fat loss happens over your entire body, and you cannot control which part of the body the fat loss comes from. The body parts that carry the most fat will be the parts that lose it last, so you must be patient. Usually it is the upper abdomen on men and the lower abdomen, hips, and thighs on women. Performing girth measurements and tracking weight over time are good ways to chart your progress. You can graph the results to keep yourself on track and analyze your results. There is no exercise that will spot-reduce a body part regardless of what is in the media. Losing fat takes a combination of nutrition, cardiorespiratory exercise, and strength training.

Following are examples of goals for fat loss:

- **Obese**: I will lose 10 pounds in the next 10 weeks by causing a weekly 3,500-calorie deficit as a result of reducing my food intake by 250 calories and increasing activity by burning 250 calories each day.
- **Overweight**: I will reduce my body fat by 1 percent over the next 30 days by performing 30 minutes of cardiorespiratory exercise three times a week at 70 percent intensity, attending a boot camp class twice a week, and eliminating sweets from my diet.

## Flexibility

Flexibility is a component of fitness that you must practice almost daily in order to see improvement, yet it is one of the most neglected parts of an exercise program. It also takes up to a year to see an improvement in flexibility; thus, you should work on your flexibility goals daily for maximum effectiveness. You can stretch after exercise or after your shower or bath while the muscles are warm.

Factors that affect flexibility include genetics and sex (typically women are more flexible than men). Younger people tend to be more flexible than older people. Other factors that affect flexibility are body shape and current level of flexibility. However, you can improve your flexibility at any age. Decide if you have a certain area or muscle on which you want to focus and use a calendar to document the number of days you stretch instead of how far you are able to stretch. This behavior goal will help you see progress over time and discourage you from doing too much too fast, which can increase the chance of injury.

By increasing your flexibility, you can improve your overall performance in activities of daily living (ADL) as well as activities done for fitness or sports. Activities of daily living include dressing, bathing, shopping, housekeeping, preparing food, and doing laundry. Fastening your seat belt requires shoulder flexibility, and putting on your socks and picking something up off the floor involve a flexible spine. Being able to take a specific joint through full range of motion can help you drive a golf ball farther or clean the shower more easily.

Following are examples of flexibility goals:

- **Young adult**: On Mondays and Wednesdays for the next three months I will participate in a yoga class at the fitness center to improve my posture and increase my joint mobility.
- **Male:** I will increase my hamstring flexibility by doing three sets of hamstring stretches in front of the TV every night during the sportscast for the next month. I will hold each stretch for 30 seconds to a point of mild discomfort.

## Balance and Core Strength

Over the past few years, improving your balance and strengthening your core have become important components of exercise programs. A strong core is critical for good balance. Keep in mind that the core is not only the rectus abdominis muscle but also all the muscles of the abdominal wall, pelvis, and lower back.

Fitness centers today have a variety of new toys that improve balance and strengthen the core. Among them are the BOSU, stability ball, balance board, and discs and foam rollers. However, you do not need fancy equipment or extra time to make improvements in your balance. Performing exercises on one leg or standing on an uneven surface while doing biceps curls improves balance. Making sure core muscles are engaged before performing a bench press improves core strength.

The following are examples of goals for balance and core strength:

- I will engage my core by contracting the pelvic floor and pulling my navel toward my spine while performing my strength training exercises for the next three workouts.
- I will improve my balance by standing on the BOSU for 15 seconds three times a week and add five seconds each week until I can balance for one full minute.

# OTHER FACTORS

Before setting your SMART goals, keep in mind four other factors. Keep in mind where you are in your fitness journey and be able to recognize road blocks. Some road blocks are foreseeable and can be dealt with, such as vacation, holiday events, and work conferences. Others cannot, such as an illness, injury, or family emergencies. You may reach a plateau where you make no progress, or you may have schedule changes.

## Motivation

Motivation is a psychological feature that stimulates you toward a goal and can reinforce a desired behavior. It compels you to act in a particular way and determines whether you will get up early for a run or sleep in. Identifying and writing down SMART goals will help you move toward a particular behavior that can motivate you to become more fit.

Not reaching a goal can discourage you and make you feel like a failure, and it can propel you back to unhealthy behavior. Understand that you can change a deadline or redo your goals—it's not an all-or-nothing situation.

## Fitness Level

In step 2 you performed a health screening and physical testing to find your weak areas and strong areas. In writing your goals, consider the areas you need to improve and the areas that you need to maintain. You may be a beginner in strength training but have excellent flexibility and balance. Or you may be able to run a marathon but cannot complete a full push-up.

Availability of fitness equipment, use of fitness facilities, and personal trainers can affect fitness goals. Decide if you should join a fitness facility or work out in your home. If you are uncomfortable exercising in front of others, go to the gym during their slow time or invest in some home equipment. Do not join a fitness center if it is not located close to home or work, and don't purchase an exercise bike if you do not like biking. You will be setting yourself up for failure.

## Social Pressures

Social influence of family and friends is another factor to consider. It is difficult to set healthy goals if your friends and family eat terribly and do not exercise. How likely are you to order a grilled chicken salad when everyone else is eating pizza and fries? Will you be able to pass up the cake and ice cream at the next birthday party? Can you continue to stay up late and still make your 6:00 a.m. spinning class? Seek out a friend or family member as a workout partner who can help the time go by more quickly than when you work out alone. When you can converse and catch up on each other's life, not only will time fly by, but you will also look forward to meeting again to work out.

Having a workout partner will also make you think twice before canceling a session because you know the other person is waiting for you at the gym. You will need to coordinate your schedules to find a time suitable to both of you, but it will help you make the time for your exercise sessions. A workout partner can also help validate how you have improved your fitness, which will help both motivation and self-esteem.

A workout partner can share in the success you are making in your progress or celebrate with you as you reach one of your goals. It is important to find the right workout partner because you might choose someone who is negative, jealous of your accomplishments, or not encouraging. It may take a few tries to find a suitable partner.

In addition to the daily influence on behavior from family and friends, the media affects our perception of what is normal. We become accustomed to seeing older people overweight and on medication, but their health problems are the result of a life of poor eating and no exercise. It is the norm only in North America, not on other continents. If you have poor eating habits and do not exercise, you will suffer the consequences and become unfit.

On the other end of the spectrum, the media also exhibits body images that are impossible to achieve and unhealthy, whether it is getting to a particular weight or size or putting on muscle to look like Mr. Olympia.

## Prioritizing Your Goals

Finally, understand how your goals will affect your work and family commitments. Finding time to start your healthy lifestyle may be challenging if you have a busy schedule. You can be creative by taking a short walk during lunch or during your break. Every minute adds up. If your evenings are chaotic, get up early and exercise. If mornings are chaotic, pack your gym bag the night before or keep workout clothes in your car. Make your goals a priority and write them in your planner just as you would a doctor's appointment.

### SUCCESS CHECK

- [x] List two barriers that may affect your goals.
- [x] List two solutions to these barriers that may affect your goals.

# REWARDS

As you reach both short- and long-term goals, it is important to reward yourself with a non-food treat. People in Western society celebrate by eating at fancy restaurants, going out for ice cream, and ordering special cakes from bakeries. Find a reward with other delights such as a massage, a new workout outfit, or a new playlist of music to accompany your workouts. This will help you feel successful, and feeling successful helps you keep on track toward your long-term goals.

# GOALS SUMMARY

Remember that getting fit is a process and includes setting goals for flexibility, balance, cardiorespiratory endurance, physical strength, and core strength and stability. You already identified your strengths and weaknesses in step 2. As you write your goals, know why you are setting them because they must relate only to you. Identify barriers and find solutions. Now that you have set your SMART goals, you will develop an action plan to help you achieve your goals and identify barriers. Above all, be ready for the unexpected, because things do happen and get in the way. Stay positive, be flexible, and don't give up.

### SUCCESS CHECK

- [x] Record what your heart rate should be in 10 weeks if you lower it by 1 beat per week.
- [x] Record the percentage of body fat you should have in 10 weeks if you lower it by 1 percent per month.
- [x] Record how much you should weigh if in 10 weeks you lose 1 pound per week.

## Before Taking the Next Step

1. Did you identify your strong and weak areas?

2. Have you written one long-term SMART goal?

3. Have you written at least three short-term SMART goals?

4. Have you included at least one behavior-oriented goal?

5. Have you included at least one result-oriented goal?

6. Did you list barriers to goals and solutions to those barriers so that you will reach your goals?

# Cardiorespiratory Exercise

Cardiorespiratory exercise, sometimes known simply as cardio or aerobics, is any form of continuous exercise lasting 10 minutes or longer that uses the large muscles of the body and increases heart rate. Cardio involves the steady and repetitive movement of the arms and legs, which makes the heart and lungs stronger.

*Aerobic* means "with air" because oxygen is necessary to accomplish the work demanded by your muscles. If you cannot get enough oxygen to the muscles (that is, if you are gasping for air), the exercise then becomes anaerobic and your duration will be short. Maximal oxygen uptake, also known as $\dot{V}O_2$max or aerobic capacity, is a good indicator of aerobic fitness level. Your $\dot{V}O_2$max tells you how efficiently your body can take oxygen from the lungs into the bloodstream and out to the working muscles. These max tests are performed in a clinical setting with a team measuring ventilation and oxygen and carbon dioxide concentrations of the exhaled air during all-out effort.

Submaximal tests estimate your cardiorespiratory fitness level and do not require an all-out effort or specialized team. They include the Cooper 12-minute walk/run test and the Rockport 1-mile walk test described in step 2.

## FACTORS THAT AFFECT CARDIORESPIRATORY FITNESS

You can improve cardiorespiratory fitness by training aerobically because the heart, like any other muscle, becomes stronger and more efficient. However, several factors affect you en route to gaining cardiorespiratory fitness: genetics, age, sex, and environmental influences.

### Genetics

Some people show improvements quickly because of good genes, while others seem to take a lot longer. The amount of oxygen your body holds is a measure of aerobic capacity. Hypertension, a disease that can be inherited, causes an increased resistance to the flow of blood, a trait that could affect the cardiorespiratory fitness of a person. Thus, you may be slower than others in gaining cardiorespiratory fitness.

## Age

Your body undergoes certain changes that affect not only your health but also your ability to perform aerobic activities. There is about a 10 percent decrease per decade in aerobic capacity as a result of the aging process in which bodily functions begin to decline. The heart and blood vessels lose elasticity and become more rigid; these processes reduce the ability to use oxygen and make the heart work harder. There is also a drop in volume of red blood cells.

## Sex

The variations in the heart structure between males and females result in differences in cardiorespiratory fitness. Men have bigger hearts with more muscle that can work harder and longer than women, so men may adapt more quickly to cardiorespiratory exercise and become conditioned more quickly; however, men are also more prone to heart disease than women. Men are typically at their peak of fitness younger in life, and women can undergo changes in fitness because of menopause.

## Environmental Influences

Besides genetics, age, and sex, you must look at your environment and lifestyle factors, because things such as alcohol use, tobacco use, drug intake, caffeine intake, stress, poor diet, environmental pollutants, and lack of exercise affect cardiorespiratory fitness. Blood volume is 95 percent water; as a result of dehydration or ingesting caffeine, your blood volume lowers and your heart has to work harder. Smoking constricts the blood vessels, increasing levels of carbon dioxide in the body and decreasing oxygen, which force the heart to work harder. Finally, as body mass increases the heart must work harder to pump blood to all the extra tissue. There are seven miles of blood vessels for every pound of body fat in your body!

Although it may seem easy for others to progress more rapidly in their fitness program, the important thing to remember is that despite good genes, age, sex, or environmental factors, it is clear that anyone can make changes in lifestyle and bring about improvements in the ability to consume oxygen and disperse it to the working muscles, thus increasing cardiorespiratory fitness. The human body is highly adaptive to aerobic endurance training.

### SUCCESS CHECK

☒ List the environmental factors that may affect your cardiorespiratory fitness and how you can decrease or eliminate these factors.

# BENEFITS OF CARDIORESPIRATORY EXERCISE

Cardiorespiratory fitness brings about numerous health benefits, most notably a decrease in risk for cardiovascular disease by 30 to 40 percent, stroke by 20 to 27 percent, type 2 diabetes, and some cancers such as colon cancer, breast cancer, lung cancer, and multiple myeloma cancers. In most cases it can lower blood pressure the same as antihypertensive medications. It enhances the immune system, which may result in fewer colds and illnesses and increases the good (HDL) cholesterol in the body.

One of the most common reasons people engage in cardiorespiratory exercise is to change body composition and lose body fat. Cardio helps you to maintain body weight or lose fat by burning calories, because once you deplete the immediate energy source (glycogen) that is stored in your muscles, you use energy (fuel) that is stored in your adipose (fat) tissue. Performing moderate cardio exercise for longer periods will burn high amounts of fat for immediate fuel needs. Shorter sessions, however, still burn large amounts fat through the afterburn effect, where your metabolism is raised hours after you perform the exercise. Cardio also increases your basal metabolic rate (the rate at which you burn calories at rest) by increasing muscle efficiency. In step 5, Muscular Strength and Endurance, you will learn more about the importance of muscle and metabolic rate in losing fat.

In addition, many internal adaptations occur with cardio conditioning, starting with a greater ability to handle intense cardiorespiratory exercise. When your heart becomes stronger, you are able to pump more blood through your veins more efficiently and rid your muscles of waste and carbon dioxide more quickly. An untrained heart may have to beat 75 to 100 times per minute, whereas a conditioned heart may have to beat only 40 to 60 times per minute to complete the same amount of work. Finally, in a well-conditioned heart, more hemoglobin in the blood and more capillaries are created, which subsequently increase the capacity to transport blood to where it is needed in the body. This allows better circulation to the brain, which can lead to improved mental acuity and memory.

Cardiorespiratory exercise releases endorphins that improve mood. Endorphins are biomechanical substances that trigger positive feelings and well-being in the body. They also reduce stress, ward off anxiety and feelings of depression, boost self-esteem, and help improve sleep patterns. You may not notice these changes immediately, but once exercise becomes part of your routine, you will notice a general sense of well-being.

### SUCCESS CHECK

☒ List three reasons you would like to benefit from performing cardiorespiratory exercise.

# FREQUENCY AND TIME

We will now discuss the recommendations, or the FITTE (frequency, intensity, time, type, enjoyment), of cardiorespiratory guidelines that are described in step 1. You will develop an understanding of where you need to start and what to include in your cardiorespiratory fitness program.

Recommendations for cardio activity vary slightly among the American Heart Association, Centers for Disease Control and Prevention, and American College of Sports Medicine. Keep in mind that a little cardiorespiratory activity is better than none, and everyone needs to start somewhere, so do not be intimidated by these recommendations. It doesn't matter if you have been a couch potato for years—you can start today by just walking. This simple change in behavior can improve your health, is easy to do, and costs nothing. You can do it anywhere with little equipment, and it's enjoyable. The important thing is to get moving!

The recommendations are to participate in 150 minutes (30 minutes 5 times per week) of moderate-intensity aerobic activity *or* 90 minutes (30 minutes 3 times per week) of vigorous-intensity aerobic activity *or* a combination of the two. In addition, if you are not yet able to perform cardiorespiratory exercise for 30 minutes, you can still earn benefits of cardio exercise if you divide your time into two or three 10- to 15-minute bouts per day. This is especially important if you have a busy schedule and cannot find the time to exercise. You can surely find 10 or 15 minutes throughout the day, possibly doing 15 minutes in the morning and 15 minutes at noon or in the evening. Research has shown this cumulative exercise can have the same effects as performing cardio all at once.

### SUCCESS CHECK

- ☒ Write down the days of the week you will be engaging in aerobic exercise.
- ☒ Write down the time (10 to 30 minutes) for each aerobic segment.
- ☒ Make sure the days and times fit in your schedule.

# INTENSITY LEVEL

Next, choose an intensity level, which is vital to the success of your program. Not measuring the intensity level of your exercise is one of the most common mistakes that beginners make. Not working hard enough can lead to lack of results and frustration, yet working too intensely can lead to burnout and injury. Moderate aerobic exercise causes a slightly increased breathing rate and provides health benefits. Intense (vigorous) aerobic exercise provides not only health benefits but also greater fat loss and a higher fitness level. We will look at three ways to monitor intensity of cardiorespiratory exercise to determine whether you are working out at a moderate pace or an intense pace.

## Talk Test

The talk test is a simple method of determining aerobic intensity if you are a beginner. No equipment or particular training is needed. With the talk test you should be able to say a sentence but not comfortably hold a conversation during exercise. If you cannot complete a sentence without taking a breath, you are working too hard; however, if you can sing while exercising, you are not working hard enough. The ability to talk throughout your cardio exercise will ensure your level of exercise is safe. Keep in mind that this method is for beginners, not advanced exercisers. As you progress in your cardiorespiratory exercise by increasing intensity, frequency, and time, you will need to make use of a different method of monitoring intensity in order to attain a higher level of cardiorespiratory fitness.

## Rating of Perceived Exertion (RPE)

This method may be the easiest and most effective way to measure exercise intensity for people of all ages, including beginners and advanced exercisers. It consists of estimating how hard you feel you are exercising both physically and mentally on a scale of 0 to 10. A rating of perceived exertion of 1 is that of a couch potato, while an

RPE of 10 is all-out exertion. Because it is individualized, it is based on your current fitness level and perception of exercise.

For most adults, an RPE of 5 to 6 is recommended, which means you should feel like you can exercise a long time; although you are breathing heavily, you can carry on a short conversation. Beginners and those with risk factors are advised to start with exercise at a rating of 3 to 4, which means breathing is easy and you can carry on a conversation. Remember to check feelings of shortness of breath as well as general level of fatigue in your muscles when you rate yourself.

RPE can be the primary method for those who have altered heart rate response or are on beta-blocker medications, which do not allow the heart rate to rise. Pregnant women would also benefit by using the RPE method because they have inconsistent energy levels and have a greater range of intensity to work with. In addition, no stops are needed in order to find a pulse or check a heart rate monitor.

### SUCCESS CHECK

☒ Choose the RPE level at which you feel most comfortable for your first three weeks of cardiorespiratory exercise.

## Target Heart Rate

The final method of determining your intensity level for cardiorespiratory exercise is target heart rate, which is also the most common method. It is a range or zone specific to your individual fitness level. There are a few steps required for calculating your ideal zone, and exercising in this zone means that you are working at a level that is intense enough to improve your cardiorespiratory fitness.

In the past we relied on the universal age-predicted method of maximum heart rate for finding target heart rate, or the formula of 220 minus age, which has a rate of error of +12 or −12 beats per minute. But you may be a fit 60-year-old, so this formula would make your target zone too low. Or you could be an out-of-shape 25-year-old who is working too hard. More recently, studies have proven a more accurate calculation in determining a target heart rate, which is the Tanaka method. Following are the four steps in calculating your intensity level when using a target heart rate range.

Once you know your target heart rate range, you can monitor it periodically throughout your workout by using a heart rate monitor worn on the wrist or chest or by manually taking a 10-second pulse check. When taking a pulse check, count the number of beats per minute starting with 0 and then multiply by 6, which will give you your beats per minute.

As you progress over time and become more fit, you will need to recalculate your target heart rate about every 2 months. If you are a beginner or have exercise restrictions because of medications, injury, or health conditions, you should be at 40 to 60 percent of your maximum heart rate. If you are an intermediate exerciser, you can work at 60 to 70 percent. If you are an advanced exerciser, you should work out at a higher range (70 to 85 percent) of your maximum heart rate. Note that if you are taking certain medications such as beta-blockers, you should not use the target heart rate formula, because the medication does not allow the heart rate to rise; thus, you may be breathing hard and sweating but the medication prevents an increase in heart rate. You will not be able to reach your target heart rate zone. Use the talk test or the

## Calculating Target Heart Rate

1. Find your maximum heart rate via the Tanaka formula:
   Max heart rate = 208 – 0.7 × age (round up the number when multiplying numbers.)

2. Subtract your resting heart rate (pulse).

3. Multiply by the range of intensity levels you choose (beginner, intermediate, advanced).

4. Add your resting heart rate (pulse).

Example: Nancy is 28 years old, has a resting pulse of 76, and is a beginning exerciser. Her intensity level will be 40 (low end) to 60 percent (high end).

28 (age) × .7 = 19.6 (round up to 20)

208 – 20 = 188, her maximum heart rate

188 – 76 (resting pulse) = 112

40% of max × 112 = 44.8 (round up to 45)

45 + 76 (resting pulse) = 121 bpm

60% of max × 112 = 67.2 (round to 67)

67 + 76 (resting pulse) = 143 bpm

Nancy's target heart rate zone is 121 to 143 beats per minute.

*Intensity for beginners is 40 to 60 percent.

RPE method of monitoring instead. And if you are on such medications, you should discuss exercise limitations with your doctor.

### SUCCESS CHECK

☒ Calculate your target heart rate zone by using the steps listed:

1. Age × .7 = _____ (round up the number)
2. Subtract from 208 = _____
3. Subtract resting pulse = _____
4. Multiply by your low end % = _____ Add resting pulse back in = _____
5. Multiply by your high end % = _____ Add resting pulse back in = _____
6. My target heart rate zone is _____ to _____ bpm

# BEST TYPES OF CARDIO

Various types of cardiorespiratory exercise include machines, aerobics classes, and recreational activities. There are a variety ways to exercise your cardiorespiratory system, and it is important to find something that suits your current health and fitness level as well as your personal preferences.

## Cardio Machines

The treadmill, stepper, elliptical, and arc trainer are cardio machines that involve your entire body weight. If you are a beginner or have health problems (obesity or joint problems), you may want to use these types of machines every other day in order to give your joints (ankles, knees, and hips) a rest. The bike, rower, seated stepper, and UBE (upper-body ergometer) machines are all performed seated, which takes the issue of body weight from the joints. Remember that all of these cardio machines work the large muscles of the body and can be effective for those at every fitness level. Cardio machines today are also very sophisticated, with ports for smart phones, tablets, and MP3 players, and they can include built-in televisions. Many have heart rate monitors and programming that ranges from walking workouts to elite race training. Some machines have optional arm movements along with leg movements.

When choosing which machines to use in your cardio program, make sure you do a variety because each machine works your muscles in a slightly different way, and each may emphasize one muscle group over another. Monday you may exercise on the treadmill (lower body), Wednesday on the rower (more upper body), and Friday on the elliptical (upper and lower body). Another option is to do 15 minutes on the stepper (lower body) and then 15 minutes on the UBE (upper body). Or 10 minutes on the treadmill (body weight); 10 minutes on the bike (seated); and 10 minutes on the stepper (body weight), which would give your joints a break in the middle of your workout.

Make sure the machine fits your body. A bike seat that is too high or too low may be uncomfortable and cause additional stress on your knees or hips, and different brands of elliptical machines have various movement ranges, which may be awkward for someone short or tall. Keep in mind cardio machines may look intimidating to new exercisers but can be very simple to use with a proper demonstration by an experienced staff member at your gym. Don't be afraid to ask for an introduction to the machines so that you're able to use them.

## Aerobics Classes

A great variety of aerobic classes are offered through organizations and fitness centers. These include hi/lo, step, boot camp, Zumba, hip-hop, interval, water aerobics, Crossfit, sport conditioning, kickboxing, and stationary cycling. New classes are continually being offered as new genres and techniques are invented. Many classes offer introductory levels. In some classes skill may be a factor, or the class may be designed for a higher level of fitness. You may want to observe a class first to see if it is something you would like to do or are able to do. Make sure the class instructor is certified by a reputable agency for safe, effective exercise. Ask for credentials.

Aerobics classes generally begin with a light aerobic warm-up and then proceed to moderate to vigorous exercises for the majority of the class. These exercises may consist of many types of movement depending on the type of class. For example, a step class is made up of rhythmic stepping moves off a six- to eight-inch platform to music. Hi/lo is the traditional type of aerobics and is either choreographed into movement combinations or freestyle. Kickboxing mimics boxing and martial arts drills, and hip-hop and Zumba classes have their own rhythm, style, and steps. Boot camp classes are simple yet intense and mimic military-style conditioning, and sport conditioning classes mimic specific sport drills using ropes, cones, and agility ladders. Water aerobics classes may be held in shallow pools where many moves are adapted from land aerobics or may be held in deep water where participants wear flotation belts. Other water aerobics classes use aquatic exercise equipment such as pool noodles, paddles, and kickboards.

All classes offered by fitness centers or organizations generally include a description of the class format and the appropriate expectations of fitness level: beginner, intermediate, or advanced. A cool-down and stretch follow, and in some classes abdominal exercises or floor exercises are included.

There are many benefits to joining a group fitness class:

- Heart-pumping music is very motivating.
- Camaraderie is a motivator—go with a friend, family member, or neighbor.
- If you find a fun class, you forget you are exercising.
- Variety keeps you from getting bored. New classes are constantly being invented.
- Social support is inspiring; class members cheer you on.
- There is not much commitment; you can try different classes until you find a good fit.
- Certified fitness instructors show modifications for exercises to accommodate your fitness level.

## Recreational Activities

Physical activities such as racket sports, basketball, and soccer can also be great types of aerobic activities. For most of these activities, you need specific skills as well as specialized equipment, fields, and teammates. Other recreational activities like swimming and outdoor cycling are not only great for any fitness level but can be done alone. These activities also require specific areas such as fields or pools and equipment. Finally, walking and running are ideal for anyone at any fitness level and can be done alone or with other participants anywhere. Remember that any activity that moves the large muscles of the body can be an aerobic exercise as long as you adhere to the guidelines for frequency, intensity, and time.

# ENJOYMENT

The last recommendation that has been added to the FITTE principle is E for enjoyment! This important detail is one that is frequently overlooked. It is essential to your long-term success that you take part in activities you enjoy. Those who participate in activities they enjoy have higher participation rates and better exercise adherence and motivation to exercise than those who choose activities they don't like. It is easy to change your unhealthy or sedentary behavior by doing something you like. If you hate to bike, do not take a cycling class. If you like music and dance, sign up for hip hop or Zumba classes. Pushed for time? Walk on the treadmill while watching a movie or a TV show. If you love basketball, do not spend 45 minutes on the stepper. Enjoyment is directly associated with retention and results.

## SUCCESS CHECK

☒   Write down three aerobic exercises you would like to include in your program that you enjoy or would like to try.

# PROGRESSION

Progression in your cardiorespiratory program depends on your starting fitness level. If you are a beginner, your cardio program should have a three-stage progression where you gradually increase the time, frequency, and intensity. These progressions are called the initial, improvement, and maintenance stages.

The initial stage, or beginning of your program, lasts about 1 to 5 months depending on your starting fitness level. Once you are able to complete 25 to 30 minutes 3 or 4 days per week at an intensity level of 60 percent, you will move on to the improvement stage. This stage can last anywhere from 6 months to 2 years depending not only on the shape you were in when you began but on all the other things that happen in life: illness, death, child rearing, relocation, military, vacation, injury, school, work. It is not uncommon to have conflicts when you are trying to reach your goals. During this stage you should be able to complete 35 to 40 minutes 3 to 5 times per week at 70 to 85 percent of your target heart rate. Finally, in the maintenance stage, you continue to exercise indefinitely. At this stage, the minimum for maintaining aerobic fitness is 3 times a week for 20 to 30 minutes at a vigorous (intense) level. A cardio log is a tool that helps you keep track of your cardio times, days, and intensity. You can use it for reaching goals or motivation as you look back to see how far you've come. Use the spaces in table 4.1 to record the types of cardio you performed, length of exercise

## Table 4.1 Sample Cardio Log

| Cardio log | Week _____ | | Date _____ | |
|---|---|---|---|---|
| Day | Activity | Duration | Level or distance | Intensity or heart rate |
| Monday | | | | |
| Tuesday | | | | |
| Wednesday | | | | |
| Thursday | | | | |
| Friday | | | | |
| Saturday | | | | |
| Sunday | | | | |

From N. Naternicola, 2015, *Fitness: Steps to success* (Champaign, IL: Human Kinetics).

bouts, distance (if you walked or ran), and intensity of exercise. Apps and websites can also store this information.

As you progress through these three stages as a beginner, increase the duration (time) before increasing the intensity level of the exercise. For example, if you start walking on the treadmill for 10 minutes at 3 miles per hour on a 0-degree incline, you would need to increase your time before increasing speed or raising the incline. Once you are able to walk 25 to 30 minutes, you can start increasing intensity by either walking faster or raising the incline. An increase in both intensity and duration is not recommended in a single session. If you can exercise in the upper range of your target heart rate zone for 24 to 30 minutes without signs of extreme fatigue for 2 to 3 weeks, you should move to the next level, because your body will adapt and the exercise will become too easy. This means you are becoming aerobically fit.

# CARDIORESPIRATORY EXERCISE SUMMARY

Cardiorespiratory exercise is important in maintaining a healthy, active lifestyle. Your program should include a variety of activities. Don't be afraid to try something new, like taking a Zumba class or entering a 5K. Make sure your program reflects your goals and time schedule. When the exercise becomes easier, increase your intensity level.

## Before Taking the Next Step

1. Did you list the days of the week (frequency) and time (duration) you will be doing cardio for the next four weeks?

2. Did you calculate or identify an intensity level for your current health and fitness level?

3. Have you decided on the best way for you to monitor your intensity?

4. Have you listed the type of cardiorespiratory exercise you will perform?

# Muscular Strength and Endurance

**M**uscular strength and muscular endurance go hand in hand and affect important parts of your daily activity that allow your body to move and to lift, push, and pull things. Muscular strength is how much weight you are able to lift in a single effort. Lifting heavy weights with low repetitions develops the fast-twitch muscle fibers, which will increase muscle mass and improve strength and power. Muscular endurance is the number of times you are able to lift the weight. Lifting lighter weights with higher repetitions develops the slow-twitch muscle fibers, which will increase muscular endurance and improve muscle tone.

## FACTORS THAT AFFECT MUSCULAR STRENGTH AND ENDURANCE

Many factors can influence muscular strength and endurance, including genetics, sex, and age. The most significant factor is genetics, which clearly plays a role in musculature (that is, muscular strength, muscular endurance, size, and appearance).

### Genetics

The type and number of muscle fibers you inherited (slow twitch and fast twitch) determine how your body will look. Training like Arnold Schwarzenegger will not produce the body of Arnold Schwarzenegger! Those with more fast-twitch muscle fibers will find it easier to gain muscle mass and strength, whereas those with more slow-twitch muscle fibers will find it easier to develop muscular endurance. Most important, you need to recognize your own characteristics and limitations to set not only practical goals but also goals that are specific to your body type and interests. For example, LeBron James would not be a good candidate for gymnastics, nor would

Gabby Douglas be a good candidate for the Olympic basketball team. In addition, some people are born with short muscles and some with long muscles. Those with long muscles are more likely than those with short muscles to develop size and strength.

## Sex

Although sex does not affect the quality of muscles, it does affect the quantity of muscles. In general, men are stronger than women because they are usually bigger, and a larger part of their total body mass is made up of muscle. However, when strength is expressed per unit of muscle fiber, men are only about 2 percent stronger than women due to larger individual muscle fibers. In addition, men have greater amounts of testosterone, which promote the growth of muscle tissue.

Women tend to be afraid of weight training because they believe they will develop big muscles. But because of low testosterone levels, they do not gain bulky muscle mass or gain significant amounts of weight unless they train intensely over many years and use some type of supplement to enhance muscle growth. Women do improve body composition, tone their muscles, and gain strength through weight training. Most untrained women who lift weights two or three days per week can gain about 1.5 pounds of muscle and lose about 3.5 pounds of fat over the first two months of weight training.

## Age

Anyone at any age can increase size, strength, and endurance of muscles, although it's easier for those to see the greatest improvement between 10 and 20 years of age. During the aging process, people lose muscle mass, which in turn makes them lose strength and endurance and makes it more difficult to perform activities of daily living. Weight training is vital to living an independent, enjoyable life as an older adult.

## Other Factors

Other factors that affect muscular strength and endurance are nutrition, rest, and design of the workout program. Not eating enough or not eating a variety of healthy protein, carbohydrate, and fat can put your body in starvation mode, so over time your body will store fat and burn muscle for energy. Step 9, Nutrition, talks about healthy eating and good food choices.

Inadequate rest (overtraining) also negatively affects development of muscles. When trying to build lean muscle with weight training, you produce microscopic tears in your muscles, and you need sufficient rest in order to repair and rebuild those muscle fibers. Proper rest will give those muscles time to heal, which is what improves your muscular strength and endurance.

Finally, the design of your workout program affects muscular strength and endurance. A weight training program that consists of a circuit of a set of 8 to 12 repetitions twice a week will result in increased fitness levels in strength and endurance. Remember that if you can't lift the weights 8 times, it's too heavy; if you can lift it 12 times easily, you should add weight. A weight training program that consists of a split routine of multiple exercises per muscle group and 3 to 5 sets of 8 to 12 repetitions 3 to 5 days a week will result in a more muscular physique. In addition, not changing your workout program over time can cause you to hit a plateau and see fewer or no results because your body adapts to the stress you place on it through your workouts. Weight training programs need to change about every 4 to 6 weeks to continually challenge your muscle tissue to perform the movement a little differently. This may involve changing the exercises, sets, reps, equipment, amount of weight, and training style.

# BENEFITS OF MUSCULAR STRENGTH AND ENDURANCE

Although most people begin weight training programs to look better, there are many other reasons you should perform weight training exercises. Besides improving your body composition (physique), you will become stronger, burn more calories, improve posture, improve bone health, reduce risk of injuries and disease, have more energy, and feel better.

No matter what type of weightlifting program you follow, whether it's an intense muscle building program or a circuit for toning the body, functional strength will increase. Everyday activities will be easier because stronger muscles can do more work, whether you are an athlete or just someone trying to open a jar of pickles. In addition, strong muscles help prevent injuries by improving balance and coordination, thus reducing the risk of falls.

Because muscle is active tissue, it burns calories 24/7. Gaining additional pounds of muscle increases your resting metabolic rate and results in a higher rate of calorie burn even when you are not exercising. In addition, a pound of muscle is more compact than a pound of fat—it takes up less space than a pound of fat, so you might lose girth before losing fat. Your weight may not change drastically in the beginning, but your physique will improve as lean muscle increases and becomes toned and fat layers become smaller. Gaining lean muscle mass makes it easier to maintain a healthy body weight.

Your posture will improve with weight training as your core, back, and shoulders become stronger. You will be able to sit or stand with a straighter back and without becoming fatigued as quickly. You will also improve bone density as the result of an increased stress placed on the bone tissue from weight training. An increase in bone density can prevent osteoporosis. Strength training may also improve joint function and positively affect insulin resistance (poor insulin resistance is associated with diabetes). Strength training also increases gastrointestinal transit time, which may be linked to colon cancer.

Energy levels throughout the day are increased for those who are more muscular because they have more stamina and don't get tired as easily. They are also able to sleep better, which can improve energy levels. Those with a lean physique may feel more confident and attractive and have more self-esteem, which can lead to a better mood.

## *SUCCESS CHECK*

ⓧ List three reasons you would personally benefit from performing weight training exercises.

# FITTE PRINCIPLE FOR MUSCULAR STRENGTH AND ENDURANCE

The frequency, intensity, time, and type of weightlifting exercises as well as the type of resistance exercises you enjoy depend on your goal: general muscular fitness, muscular endurance, muscular hypertrophy, muscular strength, or power. These aspects also affect the rate and level of strength development.

## Frequency

The recommendations for frequency in weight training depend on the volume (quantity) and intensity (quality) of the workout program and your current training status (see table 5.1). Higher volume and intense weight training require more time for muscle recovery due to microscopic tears (trauma) in the muscle, whereas less volume and lower intensity produce a smaller amount of trauma to the muscle tissue, calling for less time for muscle recovery. If you are not currently weight training or have minimal skill (beginners), you can perform 2 or 3 days per week. If you are at the intermediate or advanced level, depending on how much time you have and what best fits your schedule, you may work out 3 to 7 days per week. You may have time in your schedule for weight training 1 hour 3 days per week, or you might have time for a 30-minute workout 5 days per week. Or you may complete a 15-minute weight training circuit after your cardio workout. The important thing is to carve out time in your schedule to include weight training. Following are some examples of how muscle groups can be divided to fit the number of days of the week and the time you have available in your schedule. Keep in mind you have many combinations of muscle groups you can choose to do together, and this is just an example of how you can split up the days to accommodate your schedule:

**2 days:** Upper body and lower body
**3 days:** Chest and back, shoulders and legs, biceps and triceps
**4 days:** Chest and triceps, legs, back and biceps, shoulders
**5 days:** Chest, back, legs, shoulders, biceps, triceps

**Table 5.1  General Guidelines for Training Frequency**

| Training status | Days per week |
|---|---|
| **Beginner: not currently training or just beginning with minimal skill** | 2-3 |
| **Intermediate: basic skill** | 3-4 |
| **Advanced: advanced skill** | 4-5 |

Adapted, by permission, from T.R. Baechle, R.W. Earle, and D. Wathen, 2008, Resistance training. In *Essentials of strength training and conditioning*, 3rd ed., edited for the National Strength and Conditioning Association by T.R. Baechle and R.W. Earle (Champaign, IL: Human Kinetics), 389.

# Intensity

The recommendation for intensity is based not only on how much weight or how many sets and reps are needed in a workout but also on your training goal, as outlined in table 5.2. If you desire general muscular fitness, you can do as little as 1 set of 8 to 15 reps for each muscle group (total body) twice a week. This circuit may be ideal if you have little experience in weight training or if you don't have much time to devote to weight training. It's also an ideal place to start if you are an experienced weightlifter but have not been involved in weight training for the past six months or longer. Starting out with this circuit for the first three weeks prepares your muscles for more intense workouts and less risk of injury by allowing the connective tissue (ligaments and tendons) time to adjust to the new workload demanded from your muscles.

### Table 5.2  Recommended Intensity Based on Training Goals

| Training goal | Sets | Repetitions |
|---|---|---|
| General muscle fitness | 1-2 | 8-15 |
| Muscular endurance | 2-3 | >12 |
| Muscular hypertrophy | 3-6 | 6-12 |
| Muscular strength | 2-6 | <6 |
| Power:<br>Single-effort events<br>Multiple-effort events | 3-5<br>3-5 | 1-2<br>3-5 |

Adapted, by permission, from T.R. Baechle, R.W. Earle, and D. Wathen, 2008, Resistance training. In *Essentials of strength training and conditioning*, 3rd ed., edited for the National Strength and Conditioning Association by T.R. Baechle and R.W. Earle (Champaign, IL: Human Kinetics), 406; W.L. Westcott, 2003, *Building strength and stamina*, 2nd ed. (Champaign, IL: Human Kinetics).

## MUSCULAR ENDURANCE

If you desire muscular endurance, 2 or 3 sets and at least 12 reps are needed. Muscular endurance plays an important role in your daily activities because your muscles work all day to support your body weight. It is also important if you have to sustain an activity for long periods, carry objects, or hold a position for a long time. Increasing muscular endurance increases your stamina, so you will become less fatigued.

## MUSCULAR SIZE

Muscular hypertrophy (increased size) requires 3 to 6 sets and 6 to 12 reps. There are many reasons you may want or need larger muscles, including appearance and a corresponding increase in strength to complement functional or athletic performance. Bodybuilders require not only size but also proportion in opposing muscle groups, such as biceps and triceps, and overall upper- and lower-body proportion.

## MUSCULAR STRENGTH

If your goal is muscular strength, 2 to 6 sets and no more than 6 reps are essential. In general, all of life's physical activities involve muscular strength, including carrying groceries and getting out of your car. Muscular strength refers to the ability to lift, push, or pull against a weight. It is important to have strong muscles to help prevent injuries. Weak core muscles (low back and abdominal muscles) increase risk for low back injuries, which can lead to chronic pain.

## MUSCULAR POWER

Muscular power requires 3 to 5 sets with 1 or 2 reps for a single effort or 3 to 5 reps for multiple efforts. Those with this training goal are usually competitive athletes. Examples of muscular power are maximal jumps, sprinting, Olympic weightlifting, and exploding off the line in a football game. If power is your goal, you must be mindful of muscle gain because too much muscle can impede your performance.

## VARIETY

Remember that you should change your workout program every 4 to 6 weeks because your muscles will adapt to the exercises, resistance, and repetitions. Your body may also reach a plateau, and progress might cease if you don't change your routine.

You should make these changes by performing a variety of exercises, sets, reps, or training goals. For example, you may be interested in general fitness only, so your workout is a circuit of 8 to 10 exercises. You may keep the same protocol of doing 1 set 8 to 15 reps but change up some of the exercises or equipment. Or you may have completed 6 weeks of muscular endurance and change to 6 weeks of hypertrophy. Another example is changing the grouping of muscles worked, such as doing chest and back exercises together instead of chest and triceps. Chest and back muscles are opposing muscle groups, so when the chest is contracting, the back is stretching and vice versa. Working the chest and triceps together causes the triceps to perform additional work since they are needed during the chest exercise.

## Time

Recommendation for time (rest) between sets is influenced by your training goals and is an important part of your weightlifting program (see table 5.3). Rest allows the muscle to recover and also helps you to maintain energy levels throughout your

### Table 5.3 Rest Intervals Based on Training Goals

| Training goal | Rest |
|---|---|
| General muscular fitness | 30-90 seconds |
| Muscular endurance | ≤30 seconds |
| Muscular hypertrophy | 30-90 seconds |
| Muscular strength | 2-5 minutes |
| Power:<br>Single-effort events<br>Multiple-effort events | 2-5 minutes<br>2-5 minutes |

Adapted, by permission, from T.R. Baechle, R.W. Earle, and D. Wathen, 2008, Resistance training. In *Essentials of strength training and conditioning*, 3rd ed., edited for the National Strength and Conditioning Association by T.R. Baechle and R.W. Earle (Champaign, IL: Human Kinetics), 408; W.L. Westcott, 2003, *Building strength and stamina*, 2nd ed. (Champaign, IL: Human Kinetics).

entire workout. These short breaks range from 30 seconds to 5 minutes. However, if you are performing a strength training circuit that consists of 8 to 10 exercises and 1 set of 8 to 15 reps for each exercise, a shorter recovery time has a greater impact on the cardiorespiratory system. This may be ideal if you are trying to lose or manage weight and have less time available.

## Types of Equipment and Your Enjoyment

Recommendations on types of weight training exercises vary according to the individual and personal preference as well as the type of equipment readily available. Do you want, or have access, to use free weights, weight machines, resistance bands, medicine balls, or your own body weight? Do you want to work out at home or travel to a fitness center? What kinds of equipment or techniques do you enjoy using? You also have the option to attend a group fitness class that focuses on weight training, such as Crossfit, TRX, Les Mills BodyPump, boot camp, or sport conditioning classes. Your choice and availability of equipment should reflect your current fitness status, the time available in your schedule, your experience with weight training, and what kind of workout you really like to do.

### NONMOVEABLE MACHINES

Weight machines are pieces of equipment in which you sit, stand, or lie. The machine guides your body through the exercise as you push or pull on the resistance. They are great if you are a beginner because they are easy to use—the machine guides you through a range of motion that exhibits proper form and targets a specific muscle group, which reduces the risk of injury. They are great if you have limited time because you can progress through a workout fairly quickly: You sit on the machine and select a weight, and you don't have to load and unload weight plates or adjust to another set of dumbbells, and there's no need for a spotter to help with lifting heavy weight. Instructions posted on each machine explain not only the proper form and technique but also the muscles involved in the movement. However, the disadvantages of machines are that the machine performs the same movement through the same pattern, use few stabilizing muscles, and can become boring.

### FREE WEIGHTS

Free weights include dumbbells, barbells, pulley systems, medicine balls, kettlebells, ankle weights, and the human body—any device that can be moved freely in three-dimensional space. Compared to machines, free weights use more stabilizing muscles that support your body though the exercise. Free weights mimic more of the movements performed regularly in real life. Free weights also improve balance and coordination: It's much easier to sit and complete a chest press exercise in a machine than it is to lie on a flat bench and perform a chest press exercise using dumbbells. In addition, free weights require more brain power because they train your body to recognize where it is in space (proprioception) and whether or not it is balanced. This is important if you participate in both competitive and recreational sports.

Free weights are versatile. You can complete a variety of exercises with one set of dumbbells or a barbell or just your body weight. The disadvantage of free weights is that they take skill and proper form and technique to execute the exercise, so it's easier for your body to get out of alignment, which increases risk of injury. Free weights take more time than machines because you must load and unload weight plates. You may also need the help of a spotter to complete all the reps of a set. Most weightlifters prefer a combination of free weights and machines.

# COMPONENTS OF A MUSCULAR STRENGTH AND ENDURANCE ROUTINE

Although you may have a specific weight training goal, there are several components for all weight training programs. First and most important, beginning and intermediate exercisers should start with a 5- to 10-minute aerobic warm-up, such as walking on a treadmill or jumping rope. This allows the blood flow that is concentrated in your core to be shunted out to the extremities, thereby supplying additional blood to the working muscles to warm them up. Then perform gentle, static preexercise stretching for the muscle groups that will be worked. If you are a more advanced exerciser, active stretching (moving joints through the full range of motion) as a warm-up may be sufficient. Note that if your weight training goal is power, stretch your muscles at the end of your routine. You should perform static stretching on all muscles after resistance training. If you perform static stretching before completing power activities such as sprinting and jumping, you may impede performance.

Next, complete the weight training exercises in your program. These exercises should start with larger muscle groups followed by smaller muscle groups, because many of the smaller muscle groups are used as stabilizer (or helping) muscles. If these smaller muscles are fatigued first, the larger muscles may not be worked sufficiently. Finally, perform postexercise stretching. You have the option of stretching each muscle group after all the reps are completed for that specific muscle group or stretching all the muscles at the end of your workout.

You can perform numerous weight training exercises and combinations depending on equipment available. Following are examples of general weight training circuits where you complete exercises for the entire body in one workout as well as a split routine for a more complex weight training program in which muscle groups of the body are split and exercised on different days. The number of days depends on your schedule as well as your personal preference.

## GENERAL WEIGHT TRAINING CIRCUIT

### 8 to 10 exercises for a total-body workout in one session

- Machine leg press (glutes, quads, hamstrings): Page 105
- Multi-hip machine (abductors and adductors): Pages 109 and 111
- Machine back extension (lumbar): Page 121
- Seated cable row (lats, traps, rhomboids, rear delt, biceps): Page 79
- Machine chest press (pecs, anterior delts, triceps): Page 72
- Machine shoulder press (deltoids): Page 85
- Machine arm extension (triceps): Page 99
- Machine arm curl (biceps): Page 97
- Abdominals: Page 113

## Split Routine (2 Days)

### Day 1: Upper Body

- Chest (machine pec fly and dumbbell chest press)
- Back (lat pull-down machine and T-bar row)
- Shoulders (dumbbell lateral raise and military barbell shoulder press)
- Biceps (preacher curl and dumbbell curl)
- Triceps (cable triceps push-down and seated triceps extension)

### Day 2: Lower Body

- Glutes, quads, hamstrings (leg press machine and body-weight lunge)
- Hamstrings (hamstring curl machine)
- Quadriceps (leg extension machine)
- Abductors (side leg raise with ankle weights)
- Adductors (inner-thigh machine)
- Calves (seated calf raise and standing body-weight calf raise)

## Split Routine (3 Days)*

### Day 1: Chest and Back

- Chest (bench press, incline dumbbell press, pec fly machine)
- Back (lat pull-down, one-arm dumbbell bent-over row, body-weight pull-up)

### Day 2: Legs and Shoulders

- Legs (sled leg press, step-up, walking lunge with dumbbells)
- Shoulders (seated dumbbell shoulder press, rear delt machine, front dumbbell shoulder raise)

### Day 3: Biceps and Triceps

- Biceps (hammer curl, barbell curl, cable curl)
- Triceps (seated dip, triceps kickback, arm extension machine)

*Another combination could be chest and triceps, back and biceps, legs and shoulders. There is no wrong way to combine muscle groups.*

## Split Routine (4 Days)

### Day 1: Chest

- (bench press, flat-bench dumbbell fly, decline dumbbell chest press)

### Day 2: Legs and Biceps

- Legs (barbell squat, deadlift, seated calf raise)
- Biceps (arm curl machine, concentration curl, hammer curl)

### Day 3: Back

- (T-bar row, lat pull-down, barbell bent-over row)

### Day 4: Shoulders and Triceps

- Shoulders (shrug, incline reverse lateral dumbbell raise, machine shoulder press)
- Triceps (standing dumbbell overhead extension, cable push-down, body-weight dip)

- ☒ Identify an exercise for each body region: chest, back, shoulders, arms, legs, and core.
- ☒ List the rep range and number of sets for each exercise.
- ☒ List the exercises and equipment you are using for each muscle group.
- ☒ List the exercises in order of performance.

# PRINCIPLES OF WEIGHT TRAINING

Five principles of weight training will give you a better understanding of your weight training program and how your muscles respond to the stress (workout) you are performing. These training principles are progression, specificity, overload, reversibility, and diminishing returns.

## Progression

Progression refers to the number of repetitions performed, the number of sets completed, and the amount of weight (resistance) used. Ideally you would choose to increase one of these at a time. If your rep range is 8 to 12 and you are able to complete only 8 reps, your progression would be to lift the weight until you can do 12 reps. If your rep range is 8 to 12 and you are able to complete all 12 reps, your progression would be to increase the amount of weight. On the other hand, if you were not able to complete 8 reps with proper form and technique, decrease the weight until you are able to complete 12 full reps with proper form and technique.

## Specificity

Specificity is your muscles' adapting and responding to the specific type of stress (workout) that is placed on them. If your goal is to be better at climbing, your exercises should include the muscles and movements that mimic climbing. These would include strengthening exercises for the back, biceps, and forearms. If you would like to compete in bodybuilding you would not be successful if your workout consisted of one set of 8 to 15 reps of a circuit. On the other hand, if you are a 30-year-old businessman with a tight schedule, why would you lift weights as you did when you played high school football? Remember that your result, or outcome of your training, is specific to the stress or type of training imposed on the muscles. In addition, your muscles respond to the specific exercise that is performed and adapt accordingly.

## Overload

Overload is placing additional stress on the muscle once it adapts in order to see improvement. Without overload, your workouts would not progress and you would not see results. For example, you may start your exercise program doing 1 set of 10 reps with a 10-pound dumbbell, and it is difficult. Over time this will become easier, and if you do not place more stress on the biceps, you will see no further improvement. You can increase overload by adding more weight (such as using 12-pound dumbbells), adding another set (doing 2 sets) or increasing the reps (doing 12).

Another way to overload the muscles is changing your lifting pattern. You can do this by incorporating drop sets, negative reps, or supersets. Drop set is a technique for continuing all two or three sets of an exercise by reducing the weight once a muscle is fatigued. For example, while performing an overhead shoulder press, you may start with 30-pound dumbbells and do as many reps in proper form as you can, then drop to 25-pound dumbbells and continue performing as many additional reps as you can, then drop to 20-pound dumbbells. Negative reps involve completing additional reps after you have fatigued the muscle, with the help of a spotter. Super-sets involve working both agonist and antagonist (front and back) of a muscle with no rest in between sets. For example, work the chest and back together: After completing a set on the bench press, you immediately move to barbell rows. Supersets allow for a faster workout with multiple sets because there is no waiting or recovery time between sets. As one muscle is flexed (chest), the opposing muscle (back) is stretched. As always, stay within the guidelines of your workout program with the amount of sets and reps recommended.

## Reversibility

Reversibility is simply a concept of using it or losing it. Muscle is active tissue, and unless it is used and maintained, it will gradually shrink—you will lose the strength and endurance you worked so hard to achieve. This reinforces the importance of performing resistance training as part of your lifestyle and not as a short-term workout to get in shape. Without working out, adults lose 0.5 pound (~0.25 kg) of muscle tissue per year (10 pounds, or ~5 kg, over a 20-year period) that will affect independence and ability to perform activities. Muscular strength is lost at about half the rate it was gained, but the good news is you can gain it back with a weightlifting program.

## Diminishing Returns

The principle of diminishing returns states that genetics and sex dictate your potential for strength and muscle size. No matter how much training they perform, women cannot gain muscle the same way men can, and no matter how hard you train and eat like Arnold Schwarzenegger, you will not develop a body exactly like Arnold's.

Weight training is important to maintaining a healthy, active lifestyle. Weight training programs should reflect your goals and schedule, and you should adjust your program every 4 to 6 weeks. You have many options in adjusting a program: Change the reps or sets or the entire routine. For example, after 4 weeks of performing a general fitness circuit where you work the entire body 3 times per week, you may want to change your workout for the next 4 weeks by performing a two-day split with upper body Mondays and Wednesdays and lower body Tuesdays and Thursdays. Or you may want to keep the total-body circuit but change the exercises for each muscle group, as in performing chest presses instead of push-ups.

Another way to adjust programming is according to your schedule and activity level. If you have increased activity in the summer, you may want to spend less time weight training and do a 20-minute total-body circuit 2 days per week. If you are less active in the colder months, you may want to increase your weight training and do 45 minutes of a split routine with multiple sets per muscle group.

One of the most important days of your workout program is your day of rest. Ligaments and tendons need a break from the additional stress you are putting on your body. In addition, muscles break down and rebuild during rest. Without rest, you may find yourself overtraining, which can wreak havoc on your fitness goals.

# MOST COMMON EXERCISES

Some of the most popular exercises can be performed with or without equipment. Upper-body exercises include push-up or bench press, dumbbell row or pull-up, overhead press, biceps curl, and dip. Lower-body exercises include the squat, lunge, and calf raise. Common exercises of the core include the crunch and back extension.

## Chest

The pectoralis muscles fan over the chest area. Although the main purpose of the chest muscles is to push, they are also responsible for moving the shoulder joint and flexing and rotating the arm above the elbow. You use your chest to push a lawn mower, lift a child, arm-wrestle, and clap your hands. One of the best exercises for the chest is the push-up demonstrated in figures 5.1 and 5.2. You can perform this exercise anywhere. You can start in a modified position on your knees or in a regular push-up position on your toes.

Figures 5.1 AND 5.2    **PUSH-UP**

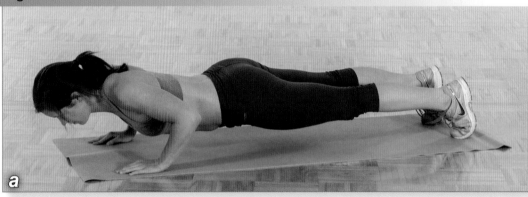

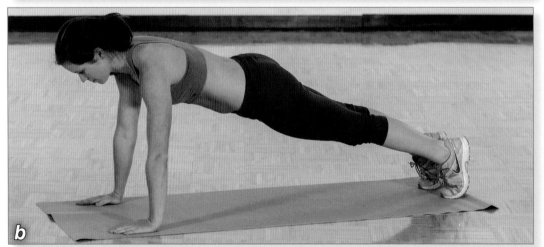

**Figure 5.1**    Proper push-up form.

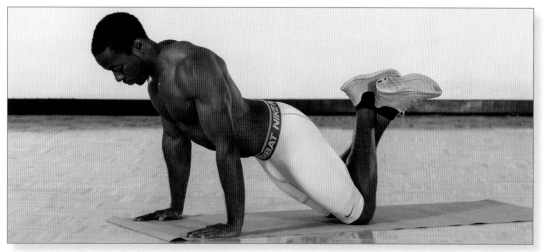

**Figure 5.2** Modified proper push-up form.

### Preparation

1. Lie facedown on the floor with your weight either on your knees (modified position) or on your toes.

2. Place your hands on the floor about shoulder-width apart. Your elbows should be pointed toward your toes.

3. Pull the navel toward the spine and relax the shoulders back and down.

### Movement

1. Exhale and slowly push up until your arms reach full range but not the locked position.

2. Your weight should be supported on your hands and knees (modified position) or toes.

3. Your spine should be in neutral alignment with your head and neck; look at the floor.

4. Inhale and lower within 4 inches of the floor, keeping your elbows close to your sides, then push back up.

*Note: Varying your hand position will affect the workout. Wider hands engage more chest muscle and closer hands engage more triceps.*

### MISSTEP
Lower back sags.

### CORRECTION
Tighten your abdominal and glute muscles.

### MISSTEP
Head drops down.

### CORRECTION
Lift your head until the back of the head is in line with the shoulders.

Figure 5.3 **MACHINE CHEST PRESS**

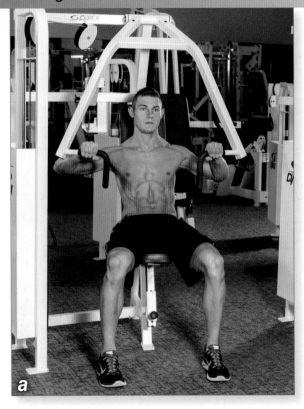

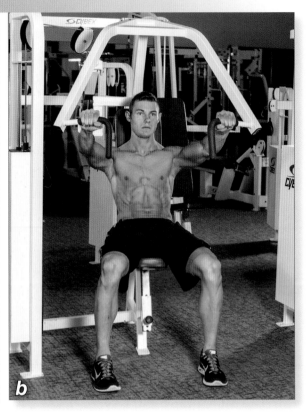

### Preparation

1. Sit in the machine with your feet flat on the floor and back and head against the padded support.
2. Grasp the handles at chest level (adjust seat accordingly).
3. Pull your navel toward your spine and relax the shoulders back and down.

### Movement

1. Exhale and slowly extend your arms until straight but not locked.
2. Keep your back and head against the pad and your wrists straight.
3. Inhale and slowly return to your starting position.

### MISSTEP
Head and neck lean forward on the push phase.

### CORRECTION
Keep chin parallel to the floor.

### MISSTEP
Weights bang together on the down phase.

### CORRECTION
Lower the weights slowly until they barely touch.

## Figure 5.4  MACHINE PEC FLY

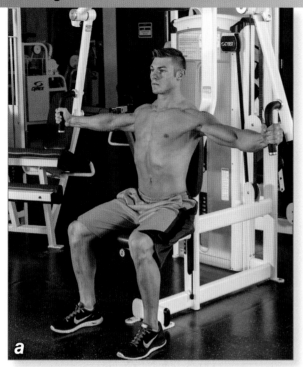
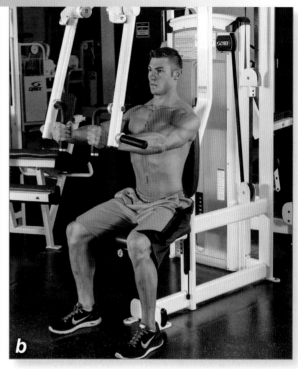

*Preparation*

1. Sit in the machine with your feet flat on the floor and back and head against the padded support.
2. Grasp the handles and extend your arms out to the side, keeping them straight but not locked.
3. Pull your navel toward your spine and relax the shoulders back and down.

*Movement*

1. Exhale and slowly bring your arms together to the front, keeping the wrists straight.
2. Inhale and slowly return to your starting position. Do not allow the arms to drift behind the body.

### MISSTEP
Head pulls forward.

### CORRECTION
Keep the head against the pad.

### MISSTEP
Shoulders round at the end of the lift.

### CORRECTION
Squeeze the shoulder blades before lifting the weight.

**Figure 5.5** **FLAT-BENCH DUMBBELL CHEST PRESS**

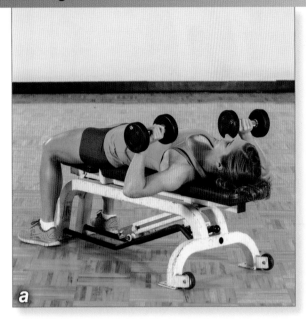

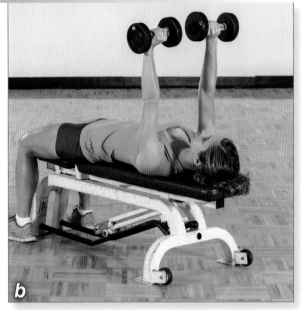

*Preparation*

1. Lie on a flat bench with a dumbbell in each hand and feet flat on the floor.
2. Position the dumbbells at the sides of the chest with palms facing forward and elbows at 90 degrees.
3. Pull the navel toward the spine and relax the shoulders back and down.

*Movement*

1. Exhale and slowly lift the dumbbells toward the ceiling until the arms are fully extended but not locked.
2. Inhale and slowly lower the dumbbells to the starting position.

**MISSTEP**

Dumbbells clang together on the upward phase.

**CORRECTION**

Control the lift so the dumbbells almost touch.

**MISSTEP**

Dumbbells are too close together on the downward phase.

**CORRECTION**

Widen the arms to 90 degrees.

Figure 5.6  **BENCH PRESS**

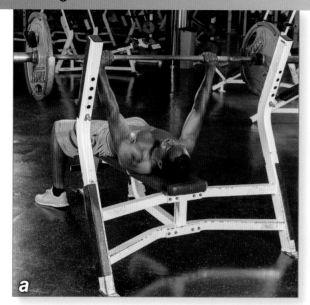
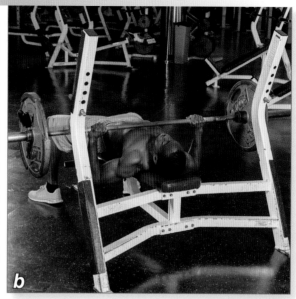

*Preparation*

1. Lie on your back with your eyes directly under the bar.
2. Place your feet on the floor and grasp the bar slightly wider than shoulder width, with palms facing forward.
3. Pull the navel toward the spine and relax the shoulders back and down.

*Movement*

1. Lift the bar off the rack and position directly over your upper chest.
2. Inhale and slowly lower the bar until the elbows are bent 90 degrees.
3. Exhale and slowly press the bar until the elbows are straight but not locked.
* Variation: Incline or decline bench may be used.

*Note: A spotter may be needed as weight increases.*

**MISSTEP**

Your low back arches off the bench or glutes lift off the bench.

**CORRECTION**

Use less weight.

# Back

The back is made up of three major muscles: latissimus dorsi, trapezius, and rhomboids. The lat muscle is the largest; it runs across the back under the armpits. It rotates the upper arm downward and inward, as in doing the downward motion of the crawl stroke in swimming. It helps pull the torso upward when climbing a ladder. The triangular-shaped trap muscle runs from the middle of the back up to the neck and across the shoulder blades. It shrugs the shoulders and lift the arms. The rhomboids squeeze the shoulder blades together and are located in the center of the back.

The main purpose of the back muscles is to pull, but they also support the neck and stabilize the torso and spine, which is necessary for good posture. Throughout the day there is constant stress on your back muscles because they are needed for sitting in a chair, getting out of the car, and carrying a heavy box. Following are two exercises that strengthen the back.

Figure 5.7    **ONE-ARM DUMBBELL ROW**

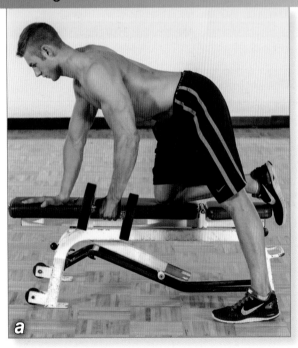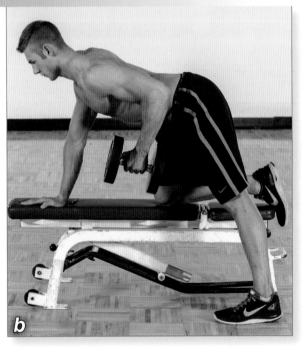

*Preparation*

1. Hold a dumbbell in your left hand.
2. Place your right knee directly under the hip on a flat bench.
3. Place your right hand directly under the shoulder on the bench.
4. Pull the navel toward your spine and keep your neck neutral.
5. Relax the shoulders back and down. Keep the shoulders even.

*Movement*

1. Exhale and slowly lift the dumbbell to your waistline without rotating the torso.
2. Inhale and slowly lower the dumbbell to the starting position without rotating the torso.

### MISSTEP
Supporting knee is too close to the supporting hand.

### CORRECTION
Place knee directly under the hip; place hand directly under the shoulder.

### MISSTEP
Shoulder rotates at the top of the lift.

### CORRECTION
Keep shoulder blades level.

### MISSTEP
Dumbbell is lifted toward the armpit.

### CORRECTION
Lift dumbbell toward your waistline.

### MISSTEP
Head and neck are lifted.

### CORRECTION
Keep eyes focused on the floor.

## Figure 5.8 LAT PULL-DOWN

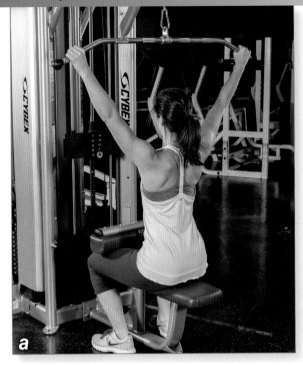

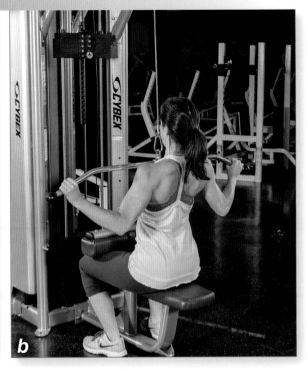

### *Preparation*

1. Sit on the machine and adjust the pad so your thighs are braced against the pad and your feet are flat on the floor.
2. Grasp the bar wider than the shoulders with the palms facing forward.

### *Movement*

1. Extend the arms, lean back slightly, and pull the shoulders back and down.
2. Exhale and slowly bring the bar to your chest, keeping the torso stable.
3. Inhale and slowly allow the bar to rise to the starting position, keeping your shoulders back and down.

---

### MISSTEP
Body leans back as the weight is pulled downward.

### CORRECTION
Keep the back and shoulders stable; toward the end of the down-ward movement, lift the chest upward to meet the bar.

### MISSTEP
Bar is lowered below the chest.

### CORRECTION
Lift the chest toward the bar on the downward phase.

## Figure 5.9 **SEATED CABLE ROW**

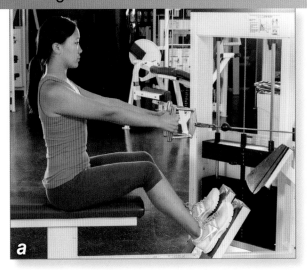
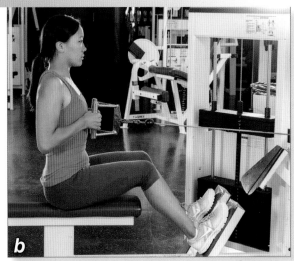

### Preparation

1. Sit on the padded seat with knees bent and feet firmly on the platform.
2. Grasp the handles, sit up tall, and relax your shoulders back and down.
3. Pull the navel toward your spine.
4. Keep your elbows close and wrists straight.

### Movement

1. Exhale and slowly pull the handles toward your belly button, squeezing the shoulder blades together.
2. Inhale and slowly return to the starting position.
3. Do not allow your shoulders to pull forward or your back to round.

### MISSTEP

Upper back rounds forward.

### CORRECTION

Pull the shoulder blades back and down and maintain throughout the lift.

Figure 5.10　**T-BAR ROW**

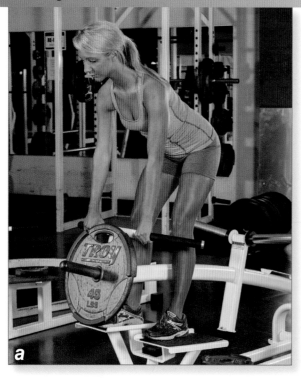 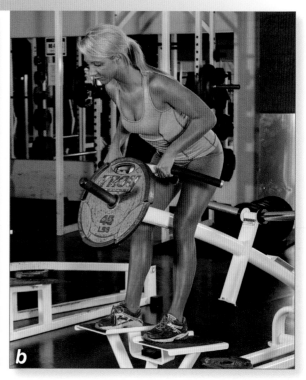

*Preparation*

1. Stand, placing your feet on the foot plate. Grasp the handles with a wide overhand grip.
2. Pull the navel toward the spine and relax the shoulders back and down.

*Movement*

1. Exhale and slowly pull the weight upward, squeezing the shoulder blades together.
2. Inhale and slowly lower the weight back to the starting position.

---

**MISSTEP**

Hyperextending chest or arching back.

**CORRECTION**

Keep back and chest flat.

**MISSTEP**

Shoulders are rounded forward.

**CORRECTION**

Keep shoulders back and down throughout the lift.

## Figure 5.11 **PULL-UP**

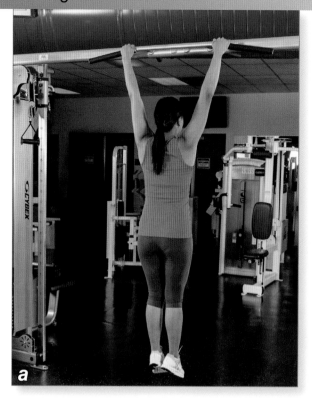
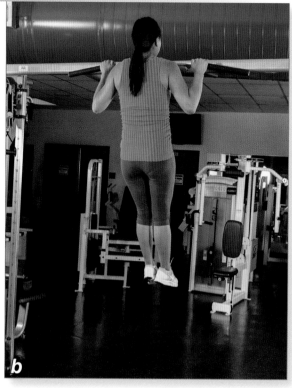

*Preparation*

1. Jump and grasp the chin-up bar with palms facing forward.
2. Pull the navel toward the spine and relax the shoulders back and down.

*Movement*

1. Exhale and slowly pull your chin even with the bar without swinging the legs.
2. Inhale and slowly lower to your starting position.

**MISSTEP**

Lower body swings during the movement.

**CORRECTION**

Keep legs crossed and pull up without momentum.

**MISSTEP**

Arms stay flexed.

**CORRECTION**

Extend arms full on the down phase.

Figure 5.12 **BENT-OVER BARBELL ROW**

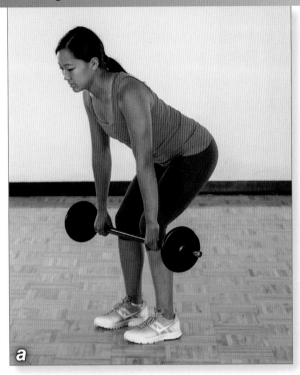
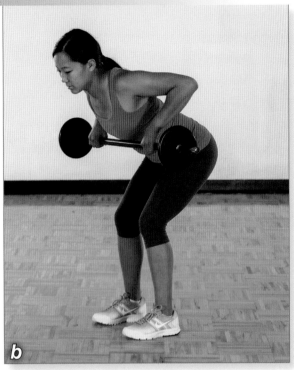

*Preparation*

1. Grasp the bar with an overhand grip, hands shoulder-width apart; lift until your hands are knee level.
2. Keep the back straight and feet shoulder-width apart; hinge from the hip.
3. Pull the navel toward the spine and relax the shoulders back and down.

*Movement*

1. Exhale and slowly lift the bar toward your navel, keeping the elbows close to your sides and pointing toward the back. Squeeze the shoulder blades.
2. Inhale and return to the starting position.

**MISSTEP**

Torso lifts up on the upward phase.

**CORRECTION**

Concentrate on keeping the back stable.

**MISSTEP**

Upper back rounds.

**CORRECTION**

Pull shoulders back and down; keep head slightly lifted.

# Shoulders

The deltoid forms the rounded part of the shoulder. This muscle stabilizes and moves the shoulder and rotates the arm. This muscle enables you to lift your arms, swing your arms while walking, and carry objects at a safe distance from the body. Following are exercises that strengthen the shoulders.

## Figure 5.13   DUMBBELL SIDE SHOULDER RAISE

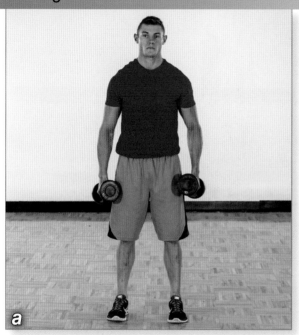
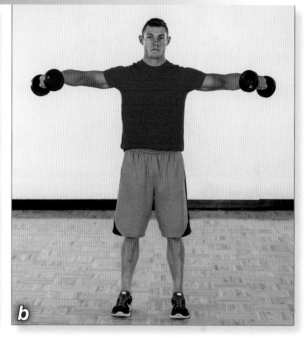

*Preparation*

1. Stand with your feet shoulder-width apart, knees slightly bent.
2. Grasp dumbbells in front of thighs, keeping your elbows slightly bent.
3. Pull the navel toward the spine and relax the shoulders back and down.

*Movement*

1. Exhale and slowly raise arms out to sides until elbows are at shoulder height.
2. Control the weight; avoid using momentum to raise the weight.
3. Inhale and slowly return to starting position.

### MISSTEP
Momentum causes the weights to fling.

### CORRECTION
Use slow and controlled movement.

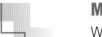

### MISSTEP
Weight is lifted too high.

### CORRECTION
Lift weight to shoulder height.

Figure 5.14　**SEATED DUMBBELL SHOULDER PRESS**

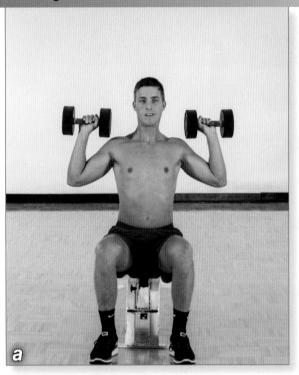

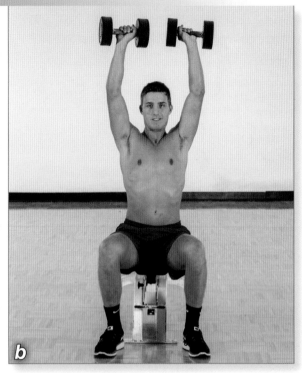

*Preparation*

1. Sit on a bench with feet flat on the floor, shoulder-width apart.
2. Hold dumbbells on each side with palms facing forward at about ear level.
3. Pull the navel toward the spine and relax the shoulders back and down.

*Movement*

1. Exhale slowly and press the dumbbells overhead until arms are fully extended but not locked.
2. Inhale slowly and return to the starting position.

**MISSTEP**

Weight is lifted directly overhead.

**CORRECTION**

Keep weight slightly in front of the face.

**MISSTEP**

Head and neck lean forward.

**CORRECTION**

Keep back straight.

Figure 5.15 **MACHINE SHOULDER PRESS**

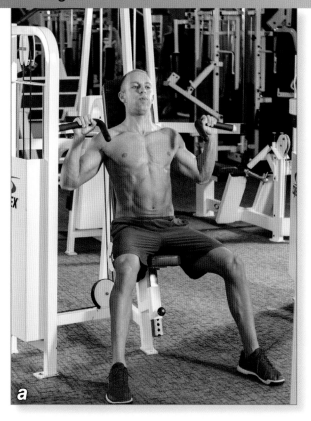

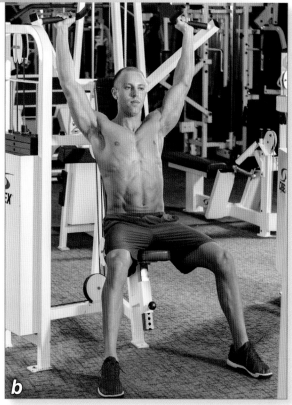

### Preparation

1. Sit with your back and head against the padded support and feet flat on the floor.

2. Grasp the handles slightly above shoulder level (adjust seat accordingly).

3. Pull your navel toward your spine and relax the shoulders back and down.

### Movement

1. Exhale and slowly lift the weight until the arms are straight but not locked.

2. Keep your back and head against the pad and your wrists straight.

3. Inhale and slowly return to starting position.

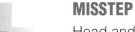

**MISSTEP**

Head and neck pull forward.

**CORRECTION**

Keep your head against the pad and chin parallel to the floor.

**MISSTEP**

Elbows lock.

**CORRECTION**

Keep a slight bend in the elbows.

## Figure 5.16 MILITARY SHOULDER PRESS

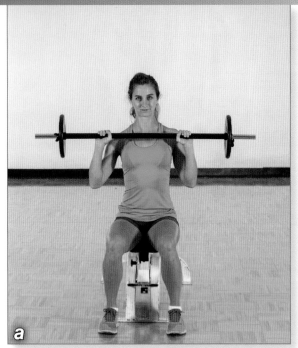

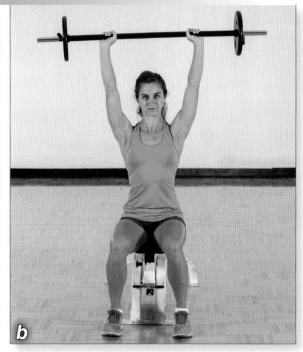

### Preparation

1. With an overhand grip, grasp a barbell slightly wider than the shoulders and lift the bar to the front of the chest.
2. Sit on a bench with your feet flat on the floor.

### Movement

1. Exhale and slowly lift the barbell overhead until the arms are straight but not locked.
2. Keep the barbell slightly in front of the face, not directly overhead.
3. Inhale and slowly lower the barbell to the starting position.

*Note: You may perform this exercise while seated or standing.*

**MISSTEP**

Torso leans forward.

**CORRECTION**

Keep your back straight.

**MISSTEP**

Elbows lock.

**CORRECTION**

Keep a slight bend in the elbows.

## Figure 5.17 STANDING BARBELL SHRUG

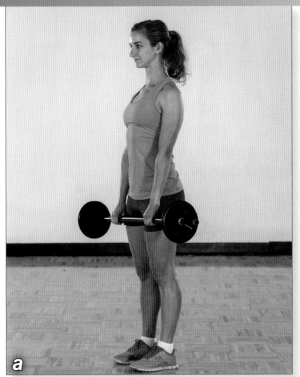
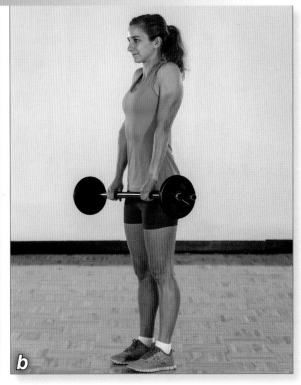

*a*

*b*

### Preparation

1. Stand with feet hip-width apart and grasp the bar with an overhand grip.
2. Position the bar in front of the thighs with the arms straight.
3. Pull the navel toward the spine and relax the shoulders back and down.

### Movement

1. Exhale and slowly shrug your shoulders upward, keeping the arms straight.
2. Do not rotate the shoulders.
3. Inhale and slowly lower the weight to the starting position.

**MISSTEP**

Shoulders rotate.

**CORRECTION**

Keep shoulders vertical throughout the lift.

**MISSTEP**

Arms bend during the lift.

**CORRECTION**

Keep arms straight.

## Figure 5.18    MACHINE REAR DELT FLY

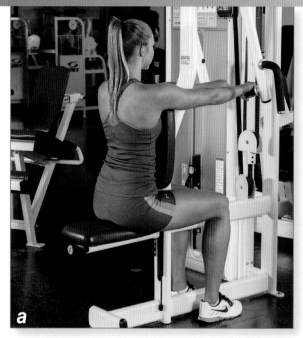 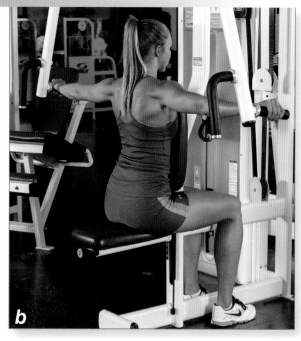

### Preparation

1. Sit on the padded support with feet on the floor, and grasp the handles at shoulder level.
2. Pull the navel in and relax the shoulders back and down.

### Movement

1. Exhale slowly and rotate your hands out to the side until they are even with the shoulders.
2. Keep arms straight but not locked.
3. Inhale and return to the starting position.
4. Do not let the weights touch.

---

### MISSTEP

Head and neck pull forward.

### CORRECTION

Keep chin parallel to the floor.

### MISSTEP

Arms fling back beyond the shoulders.

### CORRECTION

Keep the movement slow and controlled.

## Figure 5.19 INCLINE REVERSE FLY (REAR SHOULDER, UPPER BACK)

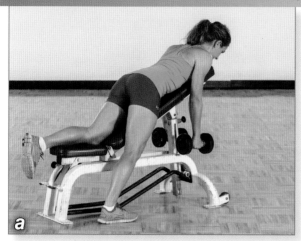
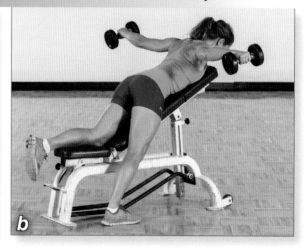

### Preparation

1. Grasp a dumbbell in each hand and lie facedown on an incline bench.
2. Extend the arms perpendicular to the bench with the palms facing in.
3. Pull the navel toward the spine and relax the shoulders back and down.

### Movement

1. Exhale and slowly lift the dumbbells until the arms are parallel to the floor; squeeze the shoulder blades.
2. Inhale and slowly return to the starting position.

**MISSTEP**
Head and neck pull forward.

**CORRECTION**
Keep neck aligned with spine.

**MISSTEP**
You use momentum.

**CORRECTION**
Pause at the top of the lift.

Figure 5.20    **FRONT DUMBBELL SHOULDER RAISE**

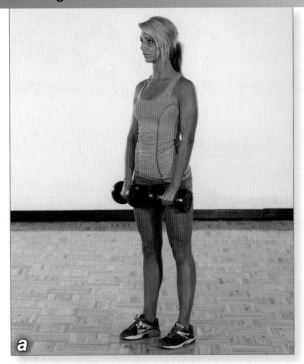

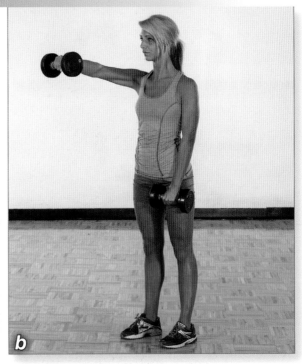

### Preparation

1. Stand with feet shoulder-width apart and knees slightly bent.
2. Place dumbbells on the front of your thighs, palms facing down.
3. Pull the navel toward the spine and relax the shoulders back and down.

### Movement

1. Exhale and slowly lift the right arm perpendicular to the floor.
2. Inhale and lower to the starting position.
3. Exhale and slowly lift the left arm perpendicular to the floor.
4. Inhale and lower to the starting position.

---

### MISSTEP
Head and neck pull forward.

### CORRECTION
Keep the chin parallel to the floor.

### MISSTEP
Elbows are locked.

### CORRECTION
Keep a slight bend in the elbow.

## Biceps

The biceps muscle is located at the front of the upper arm and is used to flex the elbow, as in picking things up or bending your elbow to scratch your nose. The biceps also rotates the forearm, as in opening a jar. Following are exercises that strengthen the biceps.

Figure 5.21　**DUMBBELL CURL**

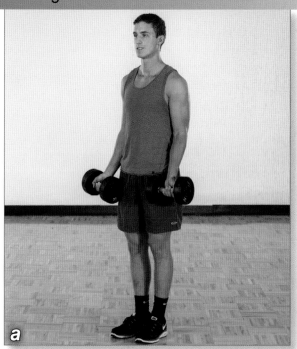 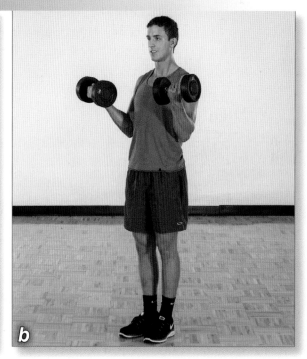

*Preparation*

1.　Stand with your feet hip-width apart and knees slightly bent.
2.　Hold a dumbbell in each hand with your arms down at your sides, palms up.
3.　Pull your navel toward your spine and relax your shoulders back and down.

*Movement*

1.　Slowly exhale and lift the dumbbells until the biceps are fully contracted.
2.　Keep the elbows pointing downward.
3.　Slowly inhale and return to the starting position.

*Note: You may also perform this exercise while seated.*

### MISSTEP

Elbows move forward.

### CORRECTION

Keep elbows pointing toward the floor.

### MISSTEP

Arms are not fully extended.

### CORRECTION

Start and finish the movement with fully extended arms.

### MISSTEP

Torso rocks forward and back during the movement.

### CORRECTION

Stand erect and tighten the core.

## Figure 5.22  HAMMER CURL

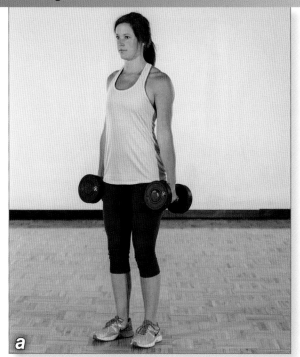
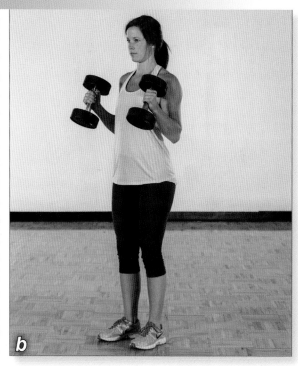

*Preparation*

1. Stand with feet hip-width apart and grasp dumbbells with palms facing inward.
2. Pull the navel toward the spine and relax the shoulders back and down.

*Movement*

1. Exhale and keep the elbows pointing downward, then slowly lift until the dumbbells are near shoulder level.
2. Inhale and slowly lower the weight to the starting position.

---

**MISSTEP**

Arms swing too far back on the downward phase.

**CORRECTION**

Control the movement and stop when the weights are at the sides.

**MISSTEP**

Arms are not fully extended.

**CORRECTION**

Start and finish the movement with fully extended arms.

**MISSTEP**

Torso rocks forward and back during the movement.

**CORRECTION**

Stand erect and tighten the core.

## Figure 5.23  CABLE CURL

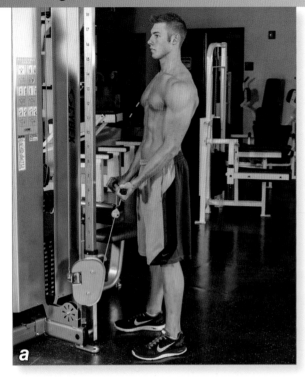

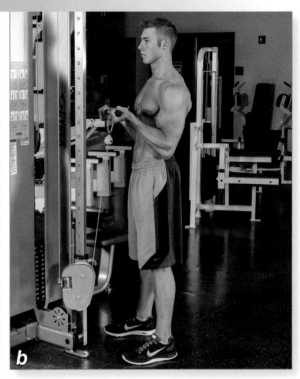

### Preparation

1. Stand near the cable pulley and grasp the bar with palms facing upward.
2. Position the feet shoulder-width apart with a slight bend in the knee.
3. Pull the navel toward the spine and relax the shoulders back and down.

### Movement

1. Exhale slowly and curl the bar until the biceps are fully contracted.
2. Keep the elbow pointing downward.
3. Inhale and slowly return to the starting position—do not allow the weights to touch.

### MISSTEP
Arms are not fully extended.

### CORRECTION
Start and finish the movement with fully extended arms.

### MISSTEP
Torso rocks forward and back during the movement.

### CORRECTION
Stand erect and tighten the core.

## Figure 5.24 CONCENTRATION CURL

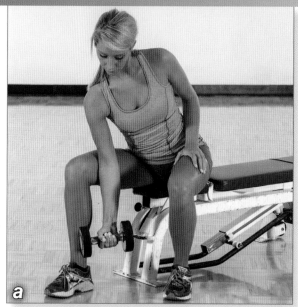

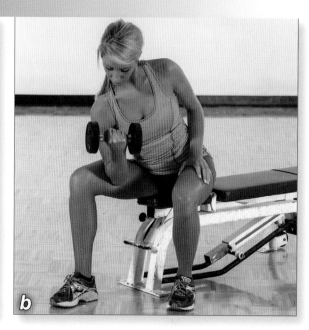

### Preparation

1. Grasp a dumbbell with the right hand and sit on a flat bench with the knees apart.
2. Place your right elbow against your inner thigh.
3. Keep your arm straight but not locked.
4. Pull the navel toward the spine and relax your shoulders back and down.

### Movement

1. Exhale and slowly curl the weight until the biceps is fully contracted.
2. Inhale and return to the starting position.
3. Grasp the dumbbell with the left hand and repeat the movement.

### MISSTEP

Upper back rounds.

### CORRECTION

Keep the back as straight as possible.

### MISSTEP

Elbow moves off the leg during the movement.

### CORRECTION

Press the elbow into the leg through the complete movement.

## Figure 5.25   PREACHER CURL

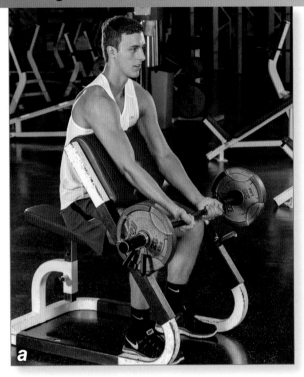

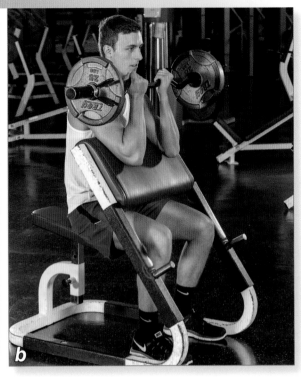

### *Preparation*

1. Grasp an EZ-bar at the close inner handle with palms facing upward.
2. Position your upper arms against the padded support and extend the arms until they are straight but not locked.
3. Pull the navel toward the spine and relax the shoulders back and down.

### *Movement*

1. Exhale and slowly lift the bar until the biceps are fully contracted.
2. Inhale and slowly lower the bar to the starting position.

### MISSTEP
Head and neck pull forward.

### CORRECTION
Keep chin parallel to the floor.

### MISSTEP
Elbows lock.

### CORRECTION
Keep a slight bend in the elbow when arms are extended.

## Figure 5.26 **MACHINE ARM CURL**

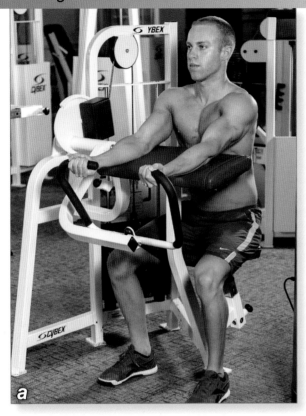
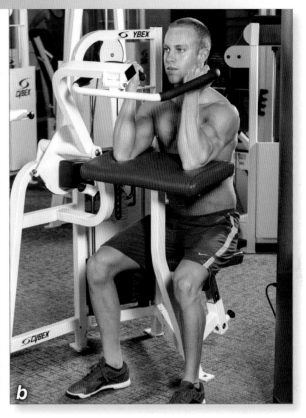

### Preparation

1. Sit in the machine with your feet flat on the floor.

2. Place your elbows slightly below the shoulders on the padded support shoulder-width apart (adjust seat accordingly).

3. Grasp the handles and make sure your elbows are aligned with the pivot point of the machine (axis).

4. Pull your navel toward your spine and relax the shoulders back and down.

### Movement

1. Exhale and slowly curl your arms upward, keeping the wrists straight.

2. Inhale and slowly return to the starting position until the arms are straight but not locked.

---

### MISSTEP

Elbows are placed too far forward on the pad.

### CORRECTION

Place elbows in line with the pivot point of the machine.

### MISSTEP

Shoulders rise during the upward phase of the movement.

### CORRECTION

Keep shoulders pressed back and down throughout the movement.

# Triceps

The triceps muscle is located at the back of the arm and is used not only to straighten the arm but also to keep the elbow from moving when performing fine movements of the forearm, such as writing. The triceps muscle is also involved in pushing actions, as in opening doors. In addition, the triceps works with other muscles to extend the arm at the shoulder joint, as when holding something behind the back. Following are exercises that strengthen the triceps.

## Figure 5.27    TRICEPS EXTENSION

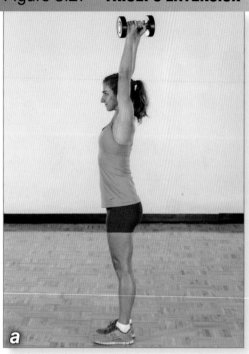 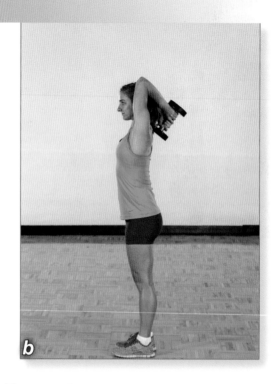

### Preparation

1. Position the feet together and keep your eyes looking forward, not down.
2. Grasp a dumbbell with both hands and lift it overhead with your arms straight but not locked.
3. Pull the navel toward the spine and relax the shoulders back and down.

### Movement

1. Keeping the elbows close to your ears, inhale and slowly lower the weight behind your head until your upper arms are perpendicular to the floor.
2. Exhale and slowly lift the weight to the starting position.
3. Keep elbows pointing upward throughout the entire movement.

*Note: You can perform this exercise seated or standing.*

**MISSTEP**

Back arches and hips rotate forward.

**CORRECTION**

Stagger the feet; tighten the core and glutes.

Figure 5.28 **MACHINE ARM EXTENSION**

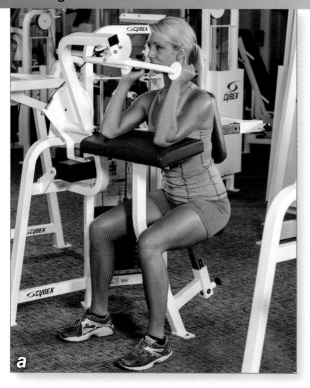
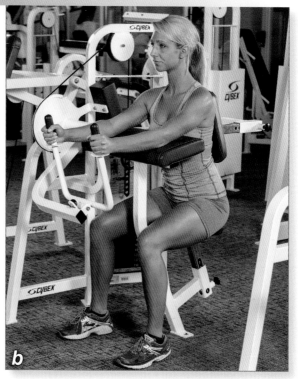

*Preparation*

1. Sit in the machine with your feet flat on the floor and back and head against the padded support.
2. Place your elbows slightly below the shoulders on the padded support shoulder-width apart (adjust seat accordingly).
3. Grasp the handles and make sure your elbows are aligned with the pivot point of the machine (axis).

4. Pull your navel toward your spine and relax the shoulders back and down.

*Movement*

1. Exhale and slowly extend your arms until straight but not locked.
2. Keep your back and head against the pad and wrists straight.
3. Inhale and slowly return to the starting position.

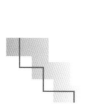

**MISSTEP**

Elbows lift off the pad.

**CORRECTION**

Push elbows down throughout the movement.

**MISSTEP**

Shoulders rise during the downward phase of the movement.

**CORRECTION**

Keep the shoulders back and down throughout the movement.

Figure 5.29 **CABLE TRICEPS PUSH-DOWN**

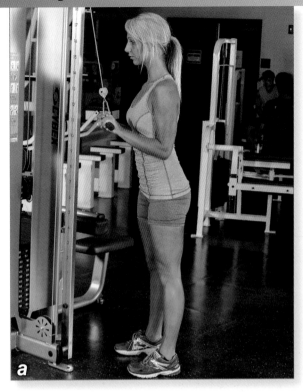

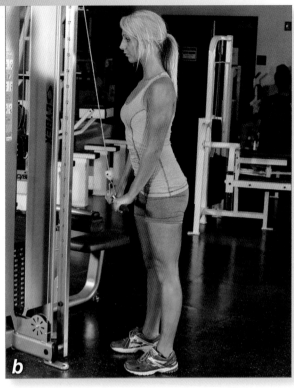

*Preparation*

1. Stand with your feet shoulder-width apart and your abdomen in. Relax your shoulders back and down.
2. Grasp the bar with hands about 8 to 12 inches (20-30 cm) apart and allow the elbows to bend more than 90 degrees.
3. Move close to the cable so that your elbows are pointing down-ward by your sides and the cable remains vertical.

*Movement*

1. Exhale slowly and push the bar down until the arms are straight but not locked.
2. Keep your elbows close to your sides and pointing downward and your wrists neutral.
3. Inhale slowly and bring the bar up to the starting position.

---

**MISSTEP**

Elbows move forward.

**CORRECTION**

Keep the elbows pointing downward.

**MISSTEP**

Bar rises too fast on the upward phase.

**CORRECTION**

Slow the movement and control the lift.

Figure 5.30 **SEATED DIP (TRICEPS)**

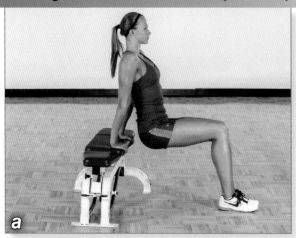
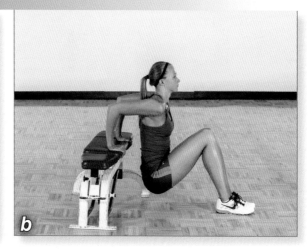

*Preparation*

1. Sit on the edge of a bench with feet flat on the floor, and place your hands so the fingertips curl over the edge of the bench.
2. Pull your navel toward your spine and relax the shoulders back and down.

*Movement*

1. Lift your butt off the bench.
2. Inhale and slowly lower until the upper arms are parallel to the floor. Keep the hips close to the bench.
3. Exhale and slowly lift until the arms are straight but not locked.

*Note: Extending the legs or placing the feet on another bench increases intensity.*

---

**MISSTEP**

Hips rock during movement.

**CORRECTION**

Keep movement in an up-and-down motion, not forward and back.

**MISSTEP**

The hips lower too far.

**CORRECTION**

Stop the movement when arms are 90 degrees.

**MISSTEP**

Arms lock or you rest at the end of the upward phase.

**CORRECTION**

Keep the elbows slightly bent.

## Figure 5.31 TRICEPS KICKBACK

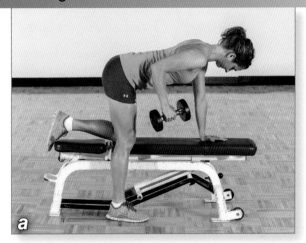
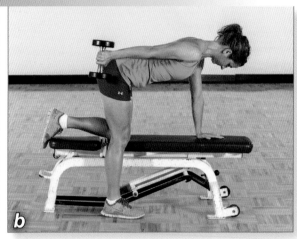

### Preparation

1. Grasp a dumbbell in your right hand and place your left knee on a bench directly under the hip.
2. Place your left hand on the edge of the bench directly under the shoulder.
3. Pull the navel toward the spine and relax the shoulders back and down. Keep the neck neutral.

### Movement

1. Lift the elbow until the upper arm is parallel and the lower arm is vertical to the floor.
2. Exhale and extend the elbow back until the lower arm is parallel to the floor.
3. Inhale and return to the starting position.

---

**MISSTEP**

Supporting knee and hand are too close.

**CORRECTION**

Place the hand under the shoulder and knee under the hip.

**MISSTEP**

Elbow moves up and down.

**CORRECTION**

Keep the upper arm parallel to the floor.

**MISSTEP**

Body and momentum fling the weight.

**CORRECTION**

Lift the weight slowly and with control; pause at the top of the lift.

# Glutes, Quads, and Hamstrings

It's difficult to isolate the glutes, quads, and hamstrings because most exercises involve all three muscle groups. The gluteus maximus is the largest, most powerful muscle in the body. The glutes extend the hip and keep the body in an upright position. The quadriceps muscle straightens the leg, and the hamstrings bend the knee and extend the hips. All are crucial in walking, running, jumping, climbing, and squatting. Here are strengthening exercises for the glutes, quads, and hamstrings.

## Figure 5.32  BARBELL SQUAT (GLUTES, QUADS, HAMSTRINGS)

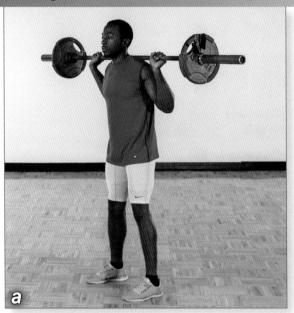

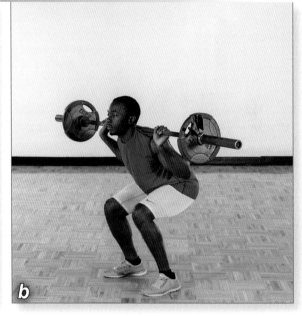

### Preparation

1. Step under the bar rack and grasp the bar wider than the shoulders with palms facing forward.

2. Position the bar low across the back of the shoulders.

3. Pull your navel toward your spine and relax the shoulders back and down; unrack the bar.

### Movement

1. With feet shoulder-width apart, inhale and slowly lower the hips back, keeping the chest up and the heels flat, until the thighs are almost parallel to the floor.

2. Do not allow your knees or ankles to roll inward or drift too far past your toes.

3. Exhale and return to the starting position, keeping your weight on your heels.

**MISSTEP**

Bar rests on your neck.

**CORRECTION**

Place the bar on your shoulders.

**MISSTEP**

Head and neck pull forward

**CORRECTION**

Keep your chin parallel to the floor, and look slightly upward.

## Figure 5.33 **SLED LEG PRESS (GLUTES, QUADS, HAMSTRINGS)**

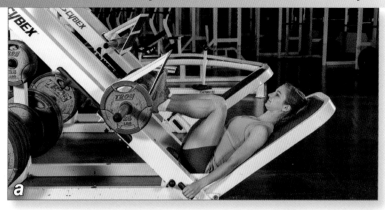

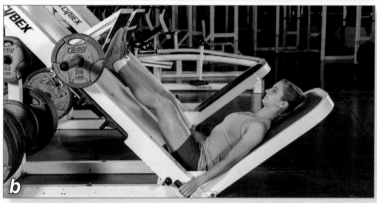

### Preparation

1. Lie on your back and place your feet hip-width apart on the platform with the toes near the top.
2. Press the weight up slightly to allow the safety bar to be released.
3. Pull the navel toward the spine, rest your head on the padded support, and relax the shoulders back and down.

### Movement

1. Inhale and slowly lower the weight until the knees are bent about 90 degrees
2. Exhale and slowly press the weight until the legs are straight but not locked.
3. To release, press the weight up slightly and engage the safety bar.

---

### MISSTEP
Head and neck pull forward.

### CORRECTION
Keep head against pad.

### MISSTEP
Knees lock.

### CORRECTION
Keep a slight bend in the knees at the top of the lift.

Figure 5.34 **MACHINE LEG PRESS (GLUTES, QUADS, HAMSTRINGS)**

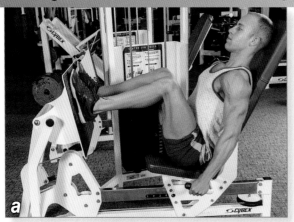
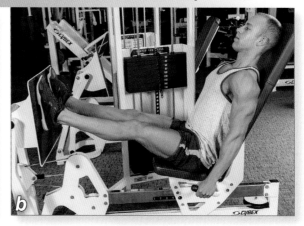

### Preparation

1. Sit on the machine with your back and head against the padded support.
2. Position your feet hip-width apart on the foot plate with knees bent about 90 degrees.
3. Feet should be flat. Grasp the handles to stabilize the upper body.
4. Make sure hips, knees, and ankles are in alignment.
5. Pull the navel toward the spine and relax the shoulders back and down.

### Movement

1. Exhale and slowly push the platform away with the heels and forefeet until the knees are straight but not locked.
2. Inhale and slowly return to the starting position, keeping the feet flat. Do not allow your thighs to compress the rib cage or let the weight plates touch.

### MISSTEP
You push the weight with your toes.

### CORRECTION
Keep your feet flat and push through your heels.

### MISSTEP
Knees move outward or inward during the movement.

### CORRECTION
Keep the knees in line with the feet and the hips throughout the movement.

Figure 5.35    **LUNGE (GLUTES, QUADS, HAMSTRINGS)**

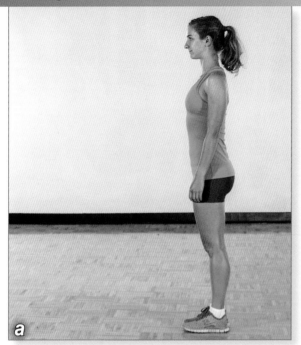

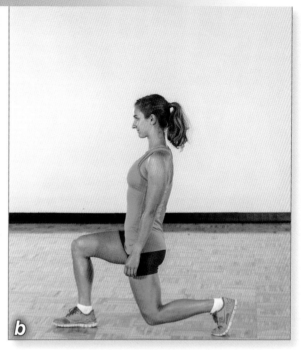

*Preparation*

1. Stand with feet together, shoulders back and down, and abs in.
2. Arms can be on your hips or by your sides.
3. Pull the navel toward the spine and relax the shoulders back and down.

*Movement*

1. Inhale and slowly lift one leg off the floor and step about 2 to 3 feet (~60-90 cm) forward.
2. Lower the hips toward the floor; knee angle should be 90 degrees.
3. Keep the back straight and avoid going too far forward; the front knee should remain behind the toes.
4. Exhale; using the heel, firmly push off the front leg to return to the starting position.
5. Repeat with the opposite leg.

*Note: You can perform this exercise with body weight, dumbbells, or barbell.*

**MISSTEP**

Your knee goes over your toe.

**CORRECTION**

Slow the movement, take a bigger step, and lower the hips.

**MISSTEP**

Torso leans forward.

**CORRECTION**

Keep the chin parallel to the floor and body erect.

Figure 5.36  **MACHINE HAMSTRING CURL**

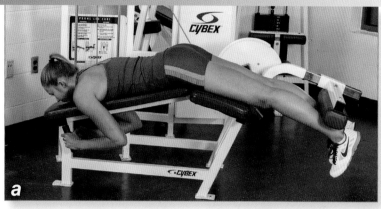

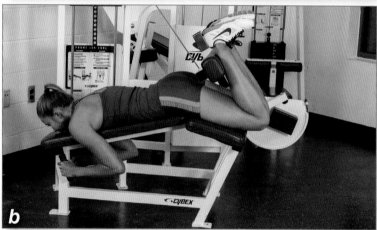

*Preparation*

1.  Lie facedown on the padded support with the leg pad a few inches above the ankle and your kneecaps off the pad.
2.  Relax the head on the pad and grasp the handles.

*Movement*

1.  Exhale slowly and curl the legs as far as possible.
2.  Inhale and slowly lower to the starting position. Do not allow the weights to touch.

**MISSTEP**

Head and neck rise.

**CORRECTION**

Rest your chin or cheek on the pad.

**MISSTEP**

Momentum causes the pad to lose contact with the back of your legs.

**CORRECTION**

Lift the weight slowly and with control; pause at the top of the lift.

Figure 5.37 **MACHINE LEG EXTENSION (QUADS)**

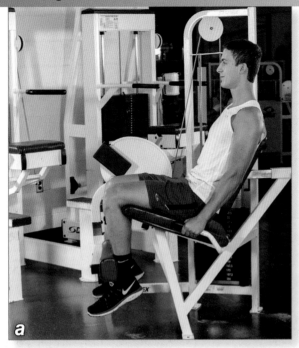
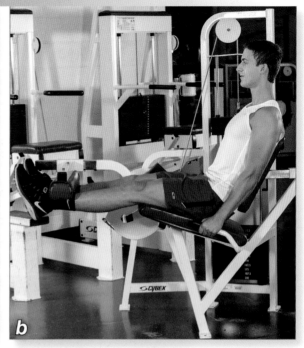

*Preparation*

1. Sit in the machine with your back against the padded support and the leg pad slightly above the ankles. Make sure the knees are aligned with the pivot point of the machine (axis).
2. Grasp the handles.
3. Pull your navel toward your spine and relax the shoulders back and down.

*Movement*

1. Exhale and slowly extend your legs until straight but not locked.
2. Inhale and slowly return to your starting position.

**MISSTEP**

Momentum causes the pad to lose contact with the front of your legs.

**CORRECTION**

Lift the weight slowly and with control; pause at the top of the lift.

**MISSTEP**

Pad is resting on the top of the feet or on the shins.

**CORRECTION**

Adjust the pad up or down so contact is slightly above the ankles.

Figure 5.38 **MACHINE HIP ABDUCTION (OUTER THIGHS)**

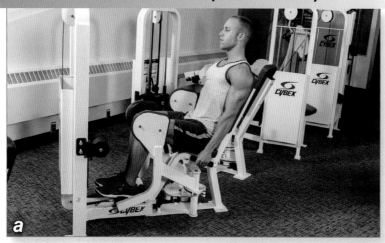

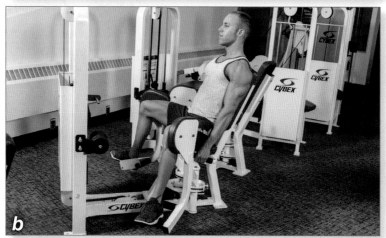

### Preparation

1. Sit on the machine with your back and head against the padded support.
2. Position your outer thighs against the pads and your feet on the support; grasp handles.
3. Pull your navel toward the spine and relax your shoulders back and down.

### Movement

1. Exhale and slowly push the thighs against the pads until you reach your full range of motion.
2. Inhale and slowly return to your starting position; do not let the weight plates touch.

**MISSTEP**

Head and neck pull forward.

**CORRECTION**

Keep head against the pad.

### MISSTEP

Momentum causes the pads to lose contact with the outer leg.

### CORRECTION

Perform the movement slowly and with control, pausing at the end of the lift.

---

**Figure 5.39  SIDE LEG RAISE (OUTER THIGHS)**

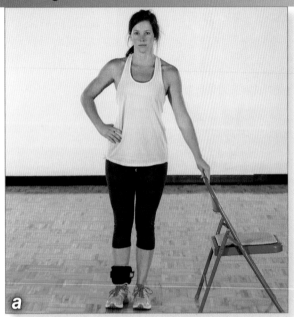
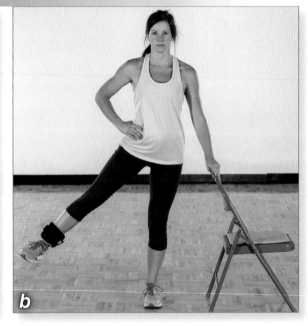

*Preparation*

1. Stand next to a chair or wall for support.
2. Pull the navel toward the spine and relax the shoulders back and down.
3. Shift your weight to the left leg, keeping a slight bend in the knee.

*Movement*

1. Exhale and slowly lift your right leg, keeping the toe and knee facing front.
2. Keep your hips level.
3. Inhale and slowly return to the starting position. Do not allow the foot to touch the floor.
4. Repeat with the weight on the right leg.

*Note: You can perform this exercise with or without ankle weights.*

---

### MISSTEP

Movement in the torso during the upward phase.

### CORRECTION

Keep the torso erect; perform the movement slowly and with control, pausing at the top of the lift.

## MISSTEP
Leg goes too high and rotates the hip.

## CORRECTION
Keep the toe and knee forward and hips level.

Figure 5.40 **MACHINE HIP ADDUCTION (INNER THIGHS)**

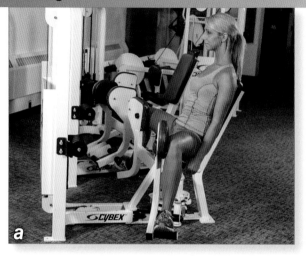
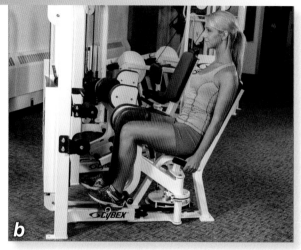

*Preparation*

1. Sit on the machine with your back against the padded support.
2. Position your inner thighs against the pads and your feet on the support; grasp handles.
3. Pull your navel toward your spine and relax the shoulders back and down.

*Movement*

1. Exhale and slowly pull the thighs together.
2. Inhale and slowly return to the starting position; do not let the weight plates touch.

## MISSTEP
Head and neck pull forward.

## CORRECTION
Keep head against pad.

## Calves

The calves allow the heels to pull up. In addition, they propel you forward when walking, running, or jumping. They also help you to climb stairs, kick a fo otball, or rise up on the balls of the feet so you can see over a fence. Following are exercises that strengthen the calf muscles.

Figure 5.41 **STANDING CALF RAISE**

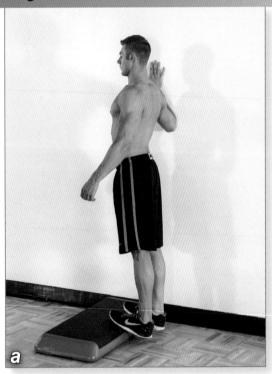
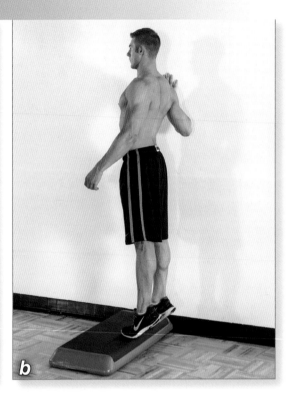

*Preparation*

1. Stand on the balls of your feet on the edge of a platform and allow your heels to drop over the edge.
2. Place your hands on a wall or chair for support.
3. Pull your navel toward your spine and relax the shoulders back and down.

*Movement*

1. Exhale and slowly rise onto the balls of the feet.
2. Inhale and slowly lower to your starting position.

*Note: You can perform this exercise on the floor.*

**MISSTEP**

Knees bend.

**CORRECTION**

Keep your knees straight but not locked throughout the movement.

Figure 5.42  **SEATED CALF RAISE**

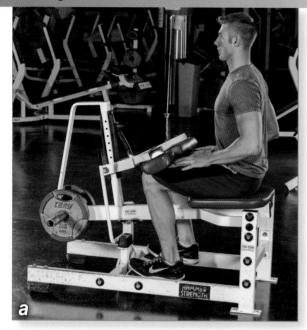 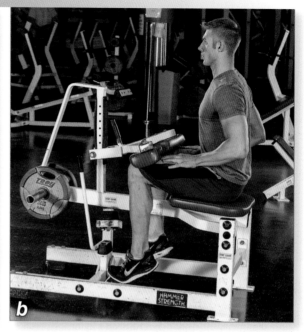

*Preparation*

1. Sit on the machine with the balls of the feet on the raised platform, and allow the heels to drop over the edge. Keep the knees aligned over the ankles.

2. Place your thighs under the lever pad and push by lifting the heels up to release the safety bar.

3. Pull the navel toward the spine and relax the shoulders back and down.

*Movement*

1. Inhale and slowly lower the heels.

2. Exhale and slowly push up onto your forefoot.

**MISSTEP**

Upper body leans forward.

**CORRECTION**

Sit erect with the chin parallel to the floor.

## Abdominals

The abdominals consist of four main groups of muscles. The rectus abdominis reaches from the pubic bone to the rib cage and moves the body between the pelvis and the rib cage. The external obliques are located on either side of the rectus abdominis and allow the torso to twist; the internal obliques are located right inside the hip-bones and move in the opposite way of the external obliques. Finally, the transversus abdominis wraps around the internal organs and stabilizes the trunk. To strengthen the abdominal muscles, you must perform exercises for each muscle group.

Figure 5.43    **AB CRUNCH (RECTUS ABDOMINIS)**

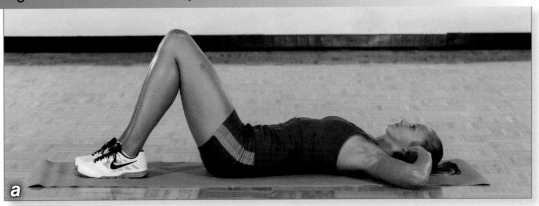

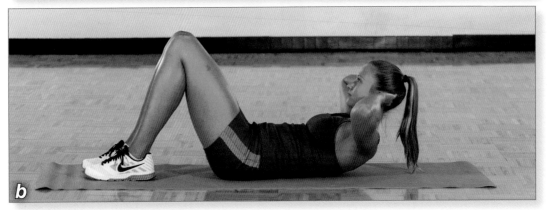

*Preparation*

1. Lie flat on the floor with knees bent about 90 degrees.
2. Pull the navel toward the spine and relax the shoulders back and down.
3. Support your head with your hands, keeping your elbows wide.

*Movement*

1. Slowly exhale and pull your rib cage toward your pelvis.
2. Keep your neck aligned and your chin off your chest.
3. Inhale and return to the starting position.

**MISSTEP**

Chin touches chest.

**CORRECTION**

Lift chin off the chest.

**MISSTEP**

Neck pulls forward.

**CORRECTION**

Keep supporting elbows wide.

**MISSTEP**

Belly pushes outward.

**CORRECTION**

Engage the transversus abdominis by pulling the navel downward.

Figure 5.44 **BICYCLE CRUNCH (INTERNAL AND EXTERNAL OBLIQUES)**

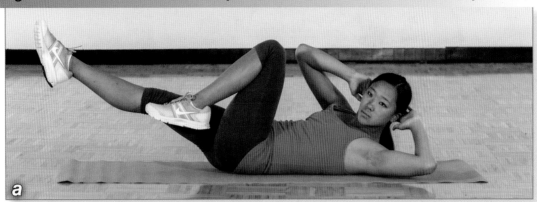

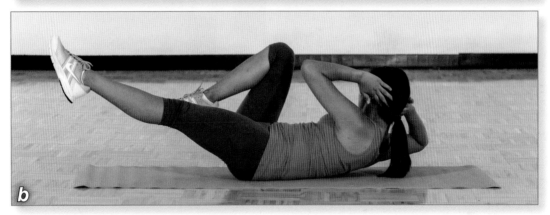

### Preparation

1. Lie on your back and support your head, keeping the elbows wide.
2. Pull the navel toward the spine and relax the shoulders back and down.

### Movement

1. Exhale and slowly bring your right shoulder toward your left knee.
2. Inhale and rotate your left shoulder toward your right knee, allowing the opposite elbow to touch the floor and the opposite leg to extend.

**MISSTEP**

Elbow touches the knee.

**CORRECTION**

Lift shoulder (not elbow) toward the knee.

**MISSTEP**

Lower back arches off the floor.

**CORRECTION**

Press navel toward the floor or eliminate leg movement.

## Figures 5.45  **MACHINE CRUNCH**

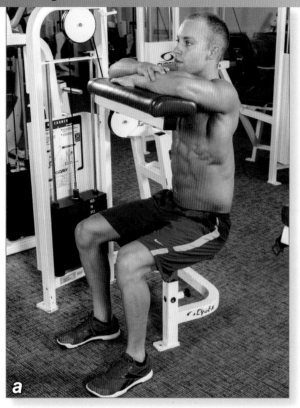

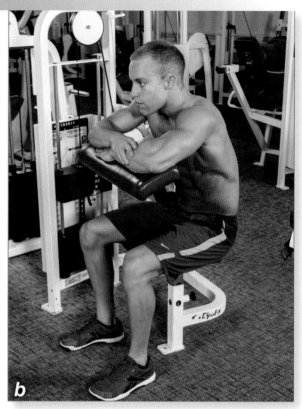

### Preparation

1. Sit in the machine with your feet flat on the floor.
2. Adjust the seat so your chin is even with the padded support.
3. Stack the forearms on the support.
4. Pull your navel toward your spine and relax the shoulders back and down.

### Movement

1. Exhale and slowly pull the rib cage toward the pelvis; do not push with your arms.
2. Inhale and slowly return to the starting position; do not let the weights touch.

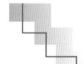

### MISSTEP

You push the pad down to the thighs.

### CORRECTION

Use the abdominal muscles, not upper body, to move the weight.

Figure 5.46 **PLANK (TRANSVERSUS ABDOMINIS)**

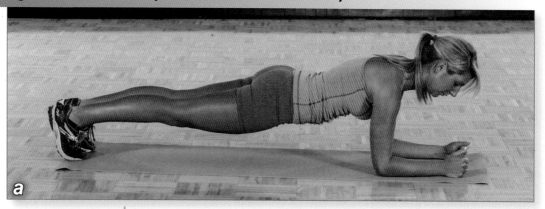

### Preparation

1. Lie on your front with your elbows directly under your shoulders and arms close to your sides.
2. Pull your navel toward your spine and squeeze the shoulders back and down.
3. Squeeze your glutes and thighs, and curl your toes under.

### Movement

1. Slowly exhale and lift your torso and thighs off the floor.
2. Do not allow your shoulders or back to sag.
3. Hold for 5 seconds or more.
4. Slowly inhale and lower to the starting position.

*Note: Modify this exercise by resting on one or both knees. It's also helpful to perform this exercise in front of a mirror to help with form.*

### MISSTEP

The low back sags.

### CORRECTION

Contract abdominal and glute muscles.

### MISSTEP

Head and neck drop downward.

### CORRECTION

Keep back of the head in line with the shoulders and hips.

# Lumbar

The muscles in the low back help support and stabilize the spine. They help you lift heavy objects and rotate the torso, which make you vulnerable to injury. Strengthening the low back muscles can prevent many types of back pain caused by too much sitting or standing. Following are exercises that strengthen the low back.

Figure 5.47 **SUPERMAN (LUMBAR)**

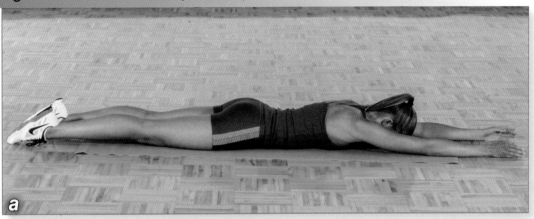

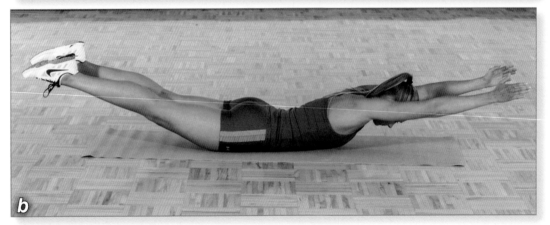

### Preparation

1. Lie facedown on a mat with both arms extended above the head, palms down, and legs straight.
2. Pull the navel toward the spine and keep your neck neutral.

### Movement

1. Exhale slowly and lift the arms and legs off the floor; hold for 5 seconds.
2. Inhale and slowly lower to the starting position.
3. Repeat on the opposite side.

**MISSTEP**

Head and neck lift up.

**CORRECTION**

Keep the eyes focused on the floor.

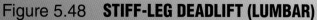

Figure 5.48 **STIFF-LEG DEADLIFT (LUMBAR)**

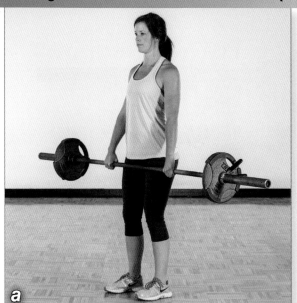

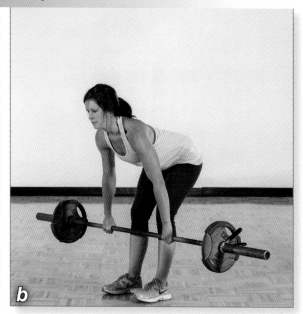

### Preparation

1. Keeping the back straight, use a shoulder-width overhand grip to grasp the barbell resting on the thighs.

2. Pull the navel toward the spine and relax the shoulders back and down.

### Movement

1. Inhale and slowly hinge from the hip and lower the weight until the bar is right below the knee.

2. Keep the knees slightly bent, back straight, and eyes looking forward.

3. Exhale and slowly return to the starting position.

**MISSTEP**

Upper back rounds.

**CORRECTION**

Hinge at the hip and keep your eyes focused forward, chin slightly up.

**MISSTEP**

Hips or shoulders move at different times.

**CORRECTION**

Move hips and shoulders simultaneously.

**MISSTEP**

Bar is too far away from the shins.

**CORRECTION**

Move bar closer to the shins.

Figure 5.49 **BIRD DOG (LUMBAR)**

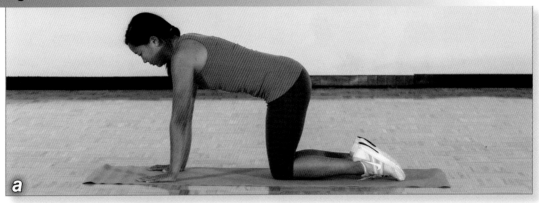

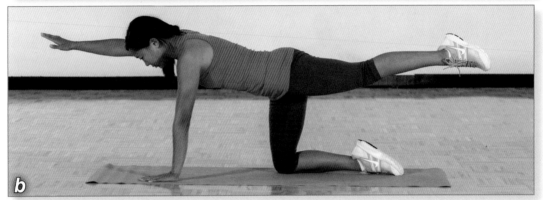

### Preparation

1. Position your hands under your shoulders and knees under your hips with fingers facing forward.
2. Pull your navel into the spine and press your shoulders back and down.
3. Keep your neck neutral.

### Movement

1. Exhale slowly and extend the right arm and left leg away from the body until they are parallel with the floor.
2. Hold for 5 seconds.
3. Inhale and slowly return to the starting position.
4. Repeat on opposite side.

*Note: Avoid excess movement and weight shifting when changing sides.*

 **MISSTEP**

Low back sags or moves during the exercise.

**CORRECTION**

Contract abdominal muscles to stabilize the low back.

 **MISSTEP**

Head and neck pull downward.

**CORRECTION**

Keep head in line with the shoulders and hips.

Figure 5.50 **MACHINE BACK EXTENSION**

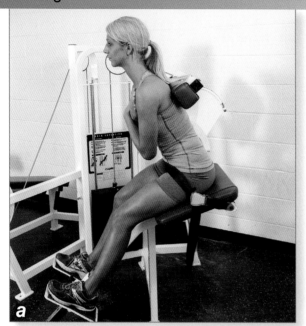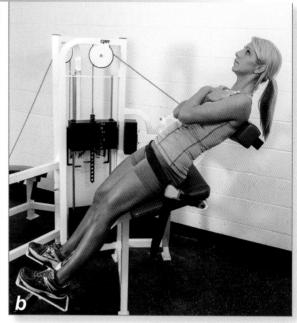

*Preparation*

1. Sit in the machine with your feet flat on the footplate and your legs extended.
2. Position the roller against the shoulder blades.
3. Make sure your hips are aligned with the pivot point of the machine (axis).
4. Fasten the seat belt (if provided) and cross the arms at the chest.

*Movement*

1. Exhale and slowly push back until the shoulders are aligned with the hips.
2. Keep the back straight.
3. Inhale and slowly return to the starting position without letting the weights touch.

*Note: Machines can vary. Follow the setup instructions listed.*

---

**MISSTEP**
Knees bend.

**CORRECTION**
Keep knees straight but not locked through the movement.

**MISSTEP**
Glutes rise from the seat.

**CORRECTION**
Use the seat belt to stay in contact with the seat pad.

# MUSCULAR STRENGTH AND ENDURANCE SUMMARY

Muscle strength and endurance are both important in maintaining a healthy, active lifestyle. Your resistance program should include a variety of exercises for each general muscle group. Design several different programs that you can use for instances when you only have 20 minutes, or you are traveling. Most of all, make sure your program reflects your goals and time schedule, and when the exercise becomes easier, make sure you increase the intensity.

## Before Taking the Next Step

1. Did you choose a weight training goal for your current health and fitness level for the next 4 to 6 weeks?

2. Did you identify the days of the week you are available for weight training?

3. Did you decide on the sets and rep range that best meet your goals for muscular strength and conditioning?

4. Did you list one or more exercises per muscle group for your workout?

5. Have you identified the equipment needed for your weight training workouts?

# Flexibility

One of the most neglected components of an exercise program is stretching to improve flexibility. Flexibility is the ability of your joints to move through a full range of motion. There are two types of flexibility but many types of stretching. Static flexibility is the ability to produce full range of motion of a joint without movement, as a gymnast demonstrates in performing a split on the floor. Dynamic flexibility is the ability to produce full range of motion during movement, as a gymnast performing a split by leaping in the air. She must use power and muscular strength to produce the flexibility, whereas a gymnast on the floor is using the floor to support the flexibility. Many types of stretching produce flexibility, as you will learn in this step.

## FACTORS THAT AFFECT FLEXIBILITY

Many factors can affect your flexibility: age, sex, joint structure, muscles, activity level, amount of adipose tissue (fat), tissue injury, and disease.

### Age

Your muscles gradually become tighter and shorter as you age, and older joints are not as healthy as younger joints. Calcium and dehydration in the joint structure increase during the aging process, and the tissue surrounding a joint has a tendency to thicken. Preadolescents are generally more flexible than adults; however, flexibility can be improved at any age but not at the same rate. Older joints take more time to develop flexibility, so older adults will need to work harder to see improvements in flexibility.

### Sex

Females are generally more flexible than males, which may be due to differences in hormone levels. Compared to men, women have more estrogen, which promotes muscle lengthening and joint laxity. Compared to women, men have more testosterone, which promotes muscle growth and shortening.

### Other Factors

The joint structure itself may also affect flexibility because of the type of joint and internal resistance within a joint, and the bony structures in a joint may limit movement. Heavily developed muscles may cause a muscle imbalance, which affects flexibility by limiting the extension of the opposing muscle group. For example, overdeveloped hamstring muscles may not allow the knee to flex to its potential. In addition, those who perform repetitive movements, whether related to a job or recreational activity, are more likely to have less flexibility in a specific joint, such as the dominant shoulder used for these activities.

Not only does inactivity result in stiff muscles and joints caused by the same chemical changes to connective tissue as aging, but sedentary individuals also tend to gain weight, which affects and inhibits mobility in joints. For example, extra fat in the abdomen may inhibit the range of motion of the hip flexors.

Muscle tissue in a joint that has been scarred due to injury decreases the elasticity of the joint. Conditions such as arthritis, bursitis, sprains, and dislocations limit the range of motion surrounding the injured body part.

### SUCCESS CHECK

☒ List the factors that may affect your flexibility.

# BENEFITS OF FLEXIBILITY

Stretching exercises that increase the range of motion throughout a joint produce many benefits. Flexibility can improve performance of daily activities, improve mobility in competitive and recreational sports, decrease the risk of injury and pain, reduce stress, and improve balance and posture.

Stretching increases blood flow to the muscles, which causes more oxygen and nutrients to be delivered to the muscle as well as waste products to be disposed. Not only does this make everyday activities easier (such as putting away groceries on the top shelf, reaching for your seat belt, or tying your shoe), but it may also help alleviate soreness.

Physical activities may be enhanced by better flexibility. If you are able to move joints through their full range of motion, muscles can produce more power, as in a baseball pitcher firing a fastball or a tennis player hitting a serve.

Flexibility indirectly helps reduce injuries. Better range of motion around a joint results in better balance; better balance means you are less susceptible to falls. Good range of motion may also reduce the trauma to a tight joint by reducing overuse injuries. For example, you may have a tight Achilles tendon, which prevents you from moving through a full range of motion when you run. Over time this can increase your risk of Achilles tendinitis. An increased range of motion may decrease microscopic tears (trauma), which not only reduces risk of injury but may also enhance performance.

Maintaining natural body alignment (posture) throughout the day is easier if you have good range of motion in your joints. Proper posture may also help prevent low back pain because stretching your low back muscles, hamstrings, hip flexors, and quadriceps helps neutralize the pelvis. Stress can cause muscles to become tense and contract, which can negatively affect areas of the body; performing stretching exercises can relax those muscles and help alleviate that stress.

# MIND–BODY EXERCISES

When it comes to fitness, most people think only about physical appearance. However, other things strongly affect the body, including stress levels, mood, and outlook on life. The mind–body connection teaches that your mind influences your body movement. Disruptions in the mind–body connection create dysfunction, which, in the fitness world, can lead to poor adherence, physical imbalances, and exercise-related injuries. In addition, how you feel about your body is directly connected with what you think about your self-worth. Thinking positive thoughts as you stretch decreases stress and calms the mind, so practicing stress-reducing exercises and mind-body techniques can improve both well-being and fitness.

These five guidelines will help you determine whether an activity is mind–body in nature:

- Focuses on breathing and breathing sounds
- Has special orientation and movement awareness
- Contains nonjudgmental sensory awareness that centers on self-reflection
- Focuses on correct postural alignment
- Involves attentiveness with the flow of movement and intrinsic energy

Mind–body practices include yoga, meditation, progressive muscle relaxation, and imagery. Yoga is perhaps the best-known exercise not only for its benefits in relaxation and flexibility but also for increasing the mind–body connection. Those who participate regularly in yoga respond more calmly to stress and have stronger parasympathetic systems, which in turn stimulate rest and relaxation in the body. You can practice yoga once a week or daily, and sessions can be short (such as performing a few poses a day) or long (such as participating in a 90-minute class). Following are several components of yoga.

## Meditation

Meditation is the art of quieting the mind to help you become more relaxed, which in turn helps the body to relax. Practicing mediation daily helps you to be more confident and more in control. It also has been known to activate the healing processes in the body. Breathe normally through your nose and close your eyes. As you exhale, choose a word or phrase, such as *I feel at peace,* and repeat several times. Repeating a word or phrase helps keep your mind focused on relaxing and not on the stresses of your day.

## Progressive Muscle Relaxation

Progressive muscle relaxation involves flexing and relaxing the muscles in a sequence, such as from head to toe, toe to head, or outer extremities (fingers and toes) toward the center of the body. Muscle groups are tensed for about five seconds and then relaxed.

## Imagery

Imagery is based on mind–body connection. It promotes relaxation and reduces stress and anxiety. Imagery uses your imagination to stimulate peace and calm to help quiet the mind. For example, close your eyes and imagine a beautiful beach and warm sand. Feel your feet sink into the sand and the warm breeze on your face. Listen to the waves crashing and see the beautiful blue water rise and fall. Many athletes use imagery to prepare for a competition.

Regardless of which method of relaxation you perform, all techniques require proper breathing as demonstrated in figure 6.1. To practice proper breathing sit or lie on the floor faceup with one hand on your abdomen and one hand on your chest. On the inhalation, let the hand on the abdomen rise as if filling a balloon. When your belly feels full of air, continue inhaling up into the chest. Exhale simultaneously from the belly and chest.

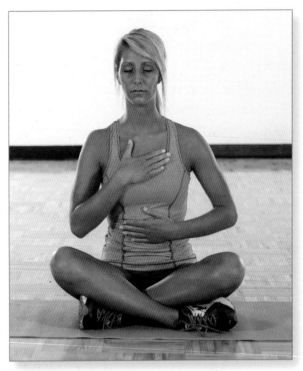

**Figure 6.1** Practicing proper breathing.

### SUCCESS CHECK

- ☒ List a mind–body exercise that you would like to incorporate into your weekly schedule.
- ☒ Choose a word or phrase to use during meditation.
- ☒ Choose a specific scene that you would find most relaxing for imagery. Practice closing your eyes and imagining a peaceful scene.
- ☒ List a sequence of muscles you would like to use in performing the progressive muscle relaxation exercise. Practice the breathing technique while either sitting or lying on the floor.

# PROGRESSION

Although your goal is to increase flexibility, it takes time, patience, and consistency to be successful. Doing too much too fast may result in a pulled muscle. Make sure you properly warm up your body, such as after cardio, after a workout, or even after taking a hot shower. Warm muscles are important in increasing flexibility.

Adding gentle movement to your stretching can help you become more flexible. Don't forget to approach stretching with caution if you have a chronic injury, because stretching a strained muscle may cause further harm.

# FREQUENCY AND TIME

Many people don't take the time to stretch, or they complain that they have limited time to exercise. Thus, they eliminate stretching from their workout plans. However, it's one of the most important and enjoyable times after a workout, especially if you have areas in your body that are tight! Stretching releases tension in the muscles developed during the workout.

If you don't have time for at least 30 minutes three times a week to stretch, take at least 5 minutes at the end of your workout to stretch. A little stretching is better than no stretching at all! You may also try doing a few stretches after a hot shower when the body temperature is elevated or while you are soaking in a hot tub. Perform a few stretches before you get out of bed in the morning by reaching your arms overhead and pointing your toes.

You should perform flexibility exercises postworkout or after a cardiorespiratory warm-up when the internal temperature of the muscle is elevated. Increased circulation brings more blood flow and warmth to the muscle, which will influence greater range of motion. Keep in mind that stretching before an intense activity such as sprinting or performances that rely on power and speed may actually result in decreased performance. Finally, don't use flexibility as a warm-up! Cold muscle fibers are more prone to injury when you stretch before exercise, and stretching is not a substitute for increasing the blood flow in a proper warm-up.

Ideally, you should stretch three to five days per week after your workouts, when you can encourage recovery and focus on rejuvenation and relaxation of mind and body. You may choose to stretch a muscle group after completing all the exercises for that muscle group or stretch at the completion of your workout. It can be time consuming to stretch regularly, but remember that unless the muscles are stretched on a regular basis, you may lose the benefits of stretching.

### SUCCESS CHECK

- ☒ Write down the days of the week you will be performing flexibility exercises.
- ☒ Write down the time in your daily routine that you would like to incorporate stretching.
- ☒ Make sure the days and times fit in your schedule.

# INTENSITY LEVEL AND TYPES OF STRETCHING

The recommended intensity level is to stretch to a point of mild discomfort, or until you feel a slight pull. Feeling pain at any time during a stretch indicates the intensity of the stretch is too high. Back off to the point where you don't feel any pain, just tension in the muscle. It's important to work within your limits—don't overdo it!

## Static Stretching

Two most common methods of stretching are static stretching and dynamic stretching. Static stretching involves coaxing a specific joint through a wider range of motion gently, not overstretching the muscle. You can use static stretching safely without equipment or assistance. For static stretching, hold the stretch for 10 to 30 seconds. Ten seconds is about three long, deep breaths. Repeat each stretch three to five times. On the exhalation, relax the muscle and sink a little deeper into the stretch. Focus on the area being stretched, limit movement in other muscles, and try to relax. Static stretching permanently increases range of motion.

## Dynamic Stretching

Dynamic stretching involves moving slowly and with control through the full range of motion and prepares the joint for full range of motion before an activity. This type of stretching is done before exercise that is movement based, such as racquetball or biking. Dynamic stretching warms up the joints, reduces muscle tension, and helps maintain flexibility. It is useful for athletes preparing for an activity involving speed. For example, before hitting the ball, a batter will swing the bat slowly through the full range of motion; or before a tennis match, a player will take a few practice swings with the racket. The key is to activate the muscles surrounding the joint with slow, controlled movement. If you use dynamic stretching inappropriately by performing the movement too fast or beyond your normal range of motion, you will incur small tears of the connective tissue in the joint.

## Ballistic Stretching

Ballistic stretching involves bouncing while holding a stretch. This type of stretching may cause small tears in the muscle, which result in scar tissue that makes the muscle less flexible and prone to pain. Although ballistic stretching may be significant in specific sport situations, the general rule is to avoid this type of stretching.

## Activated Isolated Stretching

Activated isolated stretching (AIS) is held two seconds and then released and repeated several times in a row. AIS helps the body to repair itself, especially after an injury. Using a strap or towel to assist may be helpful.

## Myofascial Release

Myofascial release uses a foam roller and your body weight to massage the fascia, or covering of the muscle. Through overuse or trauma, fascia can get tears that form scars, which can cause pain and discomfort, keeping your muscles from working the way they should. Use your body weight and roll on the foam roller until you feel a trigger point, or a painful spot. Stop and rest on the foam roller for 10 to 20 seconds. Make sure the pressure is on the muscle, not the bone or joint. This will release adhesions as well as rid the muscles of knots and tightness in your, which will increase flexibility. Although it may be uncomfortable and slightly painful, myofascial release improves mobility, function, and flexibility.

## PNF Stretching

PNF stretching, or proprioceptive neuromuscular facilitation, involves a partner using a combination of contraction and release of the muscles being stretched. Although there are various techniques in PNF, it is typically a 10-second push followed by a 10-second relaxation phase repeated several times. It is important for the facilitator to have training in administering the PNF stretching technique. PNF stretching is used not only by athletes also but by healthy adults who want to improve their flexibility.

You may also opt to participate in a stretching class such as yoga or tai chi, which may help you adhere to a stretching regimen.

# ENJOYMENT

Stretching should be safe, effective, and enjoyable! It is one of the easiest ways to relax and improve your health if you perform it correctly. How you stretch is just as important as the actual stretches. If you are not enjoying stretching, you may be straining or taking the stretch too far. If you are avoiding stretching because it is uncomfortable or you feel it is more of a chore, following are guidelines that will help you develop an enjoyable stretching routine:

- The first few days are the hardest! There may be some discomfort at first as you stretch stiff muscles that have not been stretched in a while. Don't be discouraged—it will get better as you start stretching regularly.
- Pay attention to your breathing, which will help you relax. Rather than count the seconds, try breathing deeply and slowly. Three long, deep breaths are about 10 seconds. As you exhale, relax into the stretch—it will help the muscles elongate.
- Stretch to soft music, which helps relax the mind.
- Be safe! Move slowly in and out of the stretch in the direction of the stretch. This will help prevent injuries.
- Specify an order in which you stretch, such as starting on the floor and working to a standing position, or start stretching the muscles of the upper body and work down to the lower body
- No time to stretch? You can stretch throughout the day—while standing in line, talking on the phone, doing dishes, or watching TV.
- Pay attention to your body and the movement of the muscle you are stretching. Always stretch to the point of tension or until you feel a pull, not to the point of pain.

### SUCCESS CHECK

- ☒ Write down the order of the stretches you will be performing.
- ☒ Practice each stretch with proper form.
- ☒ Check to make sure no pain is involved, only slight tension or a pull.

# STRETCHING EXERCISES

The following stretching exercises are not only easy to perform, but very effective in increasing the flexibility of muscles, ligaments, and tendons of the body. Done correctly, these exercises will increase the range of motion in your joints, which will result in easier movement and functioning throughout the day. For example, it will become easier to get out of your car, put on your jacket, or bend over to tie your shoes. Most of these exercises can be performed standing or sitting.

## Figure 6.2   CHEST EXPANSION STRETCH

The chest muscles, used for pushing, are very thick and tend to become tight quite easily, especially if you hunch forward while sitting at a desk all day or perform movements that mimic forward motion, as a house painter or hair dresser. You may find it difficult or fatiguing to sit with your back straight. Stretch your chest and front of the shoulder to improve posture and lung functioning.

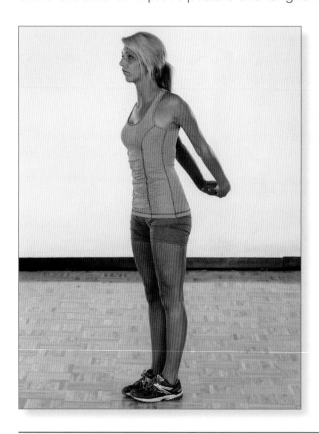

*Execution*

1. Stand with feet together.
2. Clasp hands behind the back and interlace fingers.
3. Gently press downward toward the floor.
4. Relax the shoulders and allow the chest to open.
5. Hold 10 to 30 seconds and repeat 2 or 3 times.

**MISSTEP**

Head and neck pull forward.

**CORRECTION**

Keep chin parallel to the floor.

**MISSTEP**

Elbows lock.

**CORRECTION**

Keep the elbows straight but not locked.

## Figure 6.3 UPPER BACK STRETCH

The upper back consists of a large group of muscles that help you pull and lift, movements that you perform daily. The upper-back muscles tense up more than any other part of the body, causing headache, sore shoulders, knotted back, and stiff neck. Upper-back stretches can improve posture; they have also been known to decrease stiff neck and jaw pain and relieve tension headaches. Following is a stretch for the upper back.

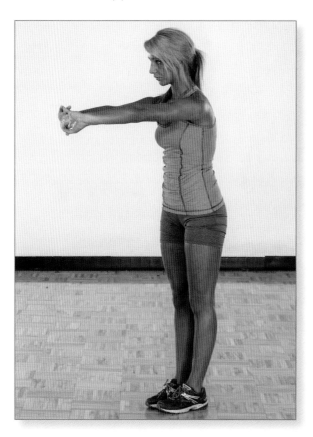

### Execution

1. Stand with feet together.
2. Clasp hands in front and interlace fingers.
3. Gently press forward.
4. Allow the upper back to round.
5. Hold for 10 or 30 seconds and repeat 2 or 3 times.

### MISSTEP
Head and neck pull forward.

### CORRECTION
Keep chin parallel to the floor.

## Figure 6.4  ONE-ARM SHOULDER STRETCH

The shoulders are one of the most neglected parts of the body. Shoulders help you with everyday tasks in reaching and lifting. Flexible shoulders improve your reaching ability and make it easier to reach your seat belt or get that high item off the top kitchen shelf. If your shoulders ache after doing some heavy lifting such as rearranging the furniture, you probably lack flexibility in the shoulders. Following is a stretch for the shoulders.

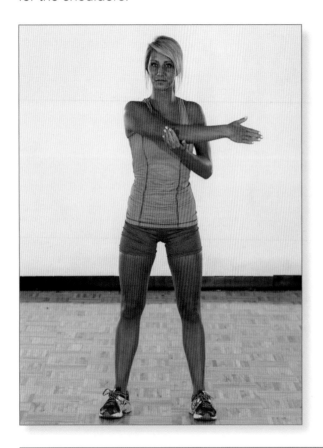

### Execution

1. Stand with feet shoulder-width apart.
2. Take the right arm across the chest.
3. Use the left arm to press the right arm gently into the chest.
4. Hold for 10 to 30 seconds and repeat 2 or 3 times.
5. Repeat with left arm.

**MISSTEP**

Shoulder lifts up.

**CORRECTION**

Keep shoulders even.

Figure 6.5 **ONE-ARM BICEPS STRETCH**

It's necessary to have normal range of motion in the biceps because they are one of the most-used muscles in the body. Movements such as opening a bottle and turning a doorknob involve the biceps. Following is a stretch for the biceps.

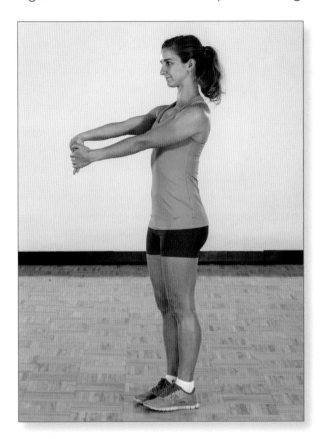

*Execution*

1. Stand with feet shoulder-width apart.
2. Extend the right arm to the front, palm facing up.
3. Use the left hand to gently press the fingers back.
4. Hold for 10 to 30 seconds and repeat 2 or 3 times.
5. Repeat with left arm.

**MISSTEP**
Elbow is bent.

**CORRECTION**
Keep elbow straight.

## Figure 6.6 ONE-ARM TRICEPS STRETCH

Triceps are the most-neglected muscles when it comes to stretching. They are also the most-underused muscles of the arm. Because they assist with shoulder movement and mobility of the arm and shoulder, you need full range of motion in the triceps. Following is a stretch for the triceps.

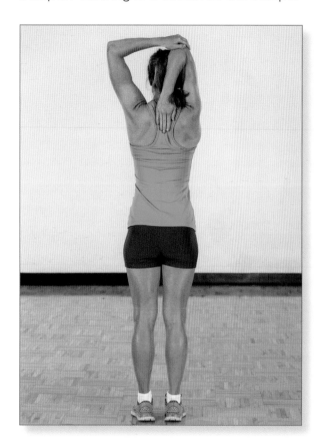

### *Execution*

1. Stand with feet hip-width apart.
2. Reach both arms overhead.
3. Allow the right hand to drop down toward the spine.
4. Use the left hand to gently pull the elbow toward the head.
5. Hold for 10 to 30 seconds and repeat 2 or 3 times.
6. Repeat with left arm.

### MISSTEP
Head and neck pull forward.

### CORRECTION
Keep chin parallel to the floor.

## Figure 6.7 ONE-LEG QUAD STRETCH

The quadriceps are bulky muscles located on the front of the thigh. These muscles extend the knee and flex the leg. Quads are the primary muscles used in walking, running, and jumping. Tight quadriceps pull on the hip bone, which pulls the pelvis forward and down, causing an arch in the low back. This arch may cause posture problems that result in low back pain. Tight quadriceps muscles may also result in weak or overstretched hamstring muscles. Sitting for extended periods shortens and tightens the quadriceps muscles, which results in a greater chance of chronic tension in the low back muscles. Following is a stretch for the quadriceps.

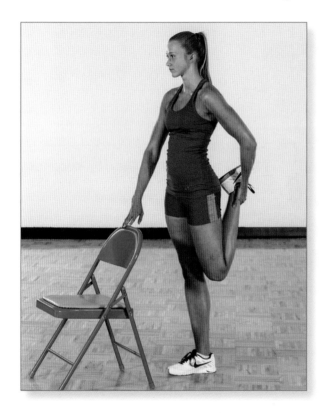

### Execution

1. Stand on the right leg, holding on to a chair or wall for support.
2. Grasp the left ankle with the left hand.
3. Lift the ankle toward the buttocks.
4. Keep the torso erect and the knee pointing downward.
5. Hold for 10 to 30 seconds and repeat 2 or 3 times.
6. Repeat with right leg.

**MISSTEP**

Torso leans forward.

**CORRECTION**

Stand erect, keeping the back straight.

**MISSTEP**

Knee is pulled backward or apart from the other knee.

**CORRECTION**

Keep knees close together and working knee pointing downward.

## Figure 6.8 SEATED HAMSTRING STRETCH

Hamstrings are located on the back of the thigh. They flex the knee and are vital for walking, running, jumping, and climbing stairs. Tight hamstrings pull on the hip bone, which pulls the pelvis backward and down, resulting in postural problems, which can lead to back pain. Many people suffer from tight hamstrings, which may be the result of sitting or driving for hours at a time. Prolonged sitting leads to shortened hamstring muscles due to the limited range of motion. Following is a stretch for the hamstrings.

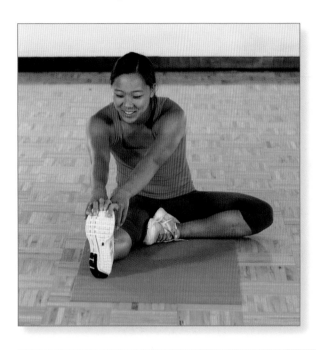

### Execution

1. Sit on the floor with one leg straight in front of you and the other leg bent to the inside.
2. Hinge forward from the hip toward the straight leg, keeping your back straight.
3. Touch the shin, ankle, or foot, whichever is comfortable for you.
4. Do not allow the knee to bend.
5. Hold for 10 to 30 seconds and repeat 2 or 3 times.
6. Repeat with right leg.

### MISSTEP
Front leg bends.

### CORRECTION
Keep leg straight but not locked.

### MISSTEP
Upper back rounds.

### CORRECTION
Keep back straight, chin parallel with the floor.

## Figure 6.9 LYING HIP STRETCH

Tight hips and outer thighs seem to be a widespread problem for many people. Tight hips may alter the position of the leg, causing an uneven distribution of forces through the knee when you walk or run. It may also limit pelvic mobility, which can cause back pain and stiffness. In addition, the muscles of the outer hip can be overactive, causing additional compromised pelvic motion. Following is a stretch for the hips and outer thigh.

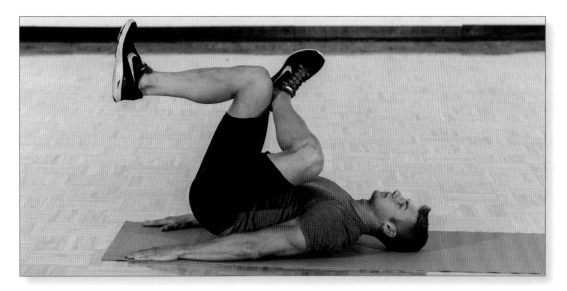

### Execution

1. Lie down with knees bent.
2. Cross the left leg over the right knee.
3. Lift both knees toward the chest.
4. Hold for 10 to 30 seconds and repeat 2 or 3 times.
5. Repeat, crossing the right leg over the left knee.

### MISSTEP
Head lifts off the floor.

### CORRECTION
Keep head rested against the floor.

## Figure 6.10  SEATED INNER THIGH STRETCH

Tight muscles of the inner thigh can cause the upper leg to rotate inward, which can cause knee pain. Tight inner thighs also cannot stabilize the knee when running, so the hamstrings must engage to assist, putting them at a higher risk of injury. Following is a stretch for the inner thighs.

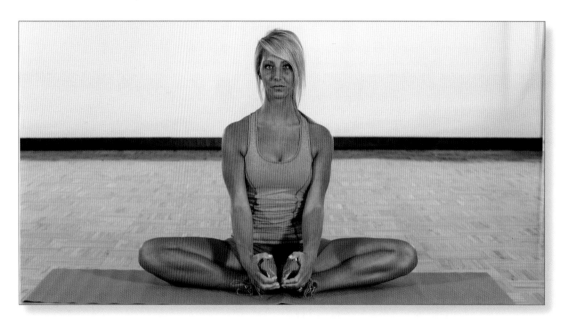

### Execution

1. Sit with soles of feet together.
2. Grasp feet with hands.
3. Slowly lean forward until you feel a pull.
4. Hold for 10 to 30 seconds and repeat 2 or 3 times.

---

### MISSTEP
Upper back rounds.

### CORRECTION
Keep back straight and chin parallel to the floor.

## Figure 6.11    CALF STRETCH AGAINST A WALL

Tight calf muscles are a common complaint because so many daily movements are oriented toward activating and shortening the calf muscle, and this can limit foot and ankle range of motion, which in turn affects walking and running gait. Tight calves can lead to chronic pain in the Achilles tendon and result in plantar fasciitis and shin splints. Wearing high heels can shorten the calf muscle and also lead to plantar fasciitis as well as foot and ankle problems. Following is a stretch for the calf muscles.

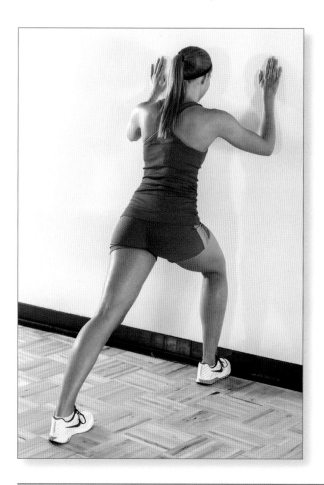

### Execution

1. Stand and place both hands on a wall.
2. Extend the left leg back.
3. Gently press the heel to the floor until you feel a pull.
4. Keep your back straight.
5. Hold for 10 to 30 seconds and repeat 2 or 3 times.
6. Repeat on the other side.

### MISSTEP
Back heel is off the floor.

### CORRECTION
Move closer to the wall.

## Figure 6.12   HIP FLEXOR STRETCH

Tight hip flexors correspond with tight quadriceps, which leads to a forward pelvic tilt and increases the curve in the low back, resulting in low back pain. Tight hip flexors are caused by being in a seated position for extended periods. Following is a stretch for the hip flexors.

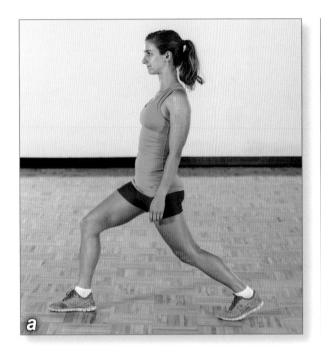

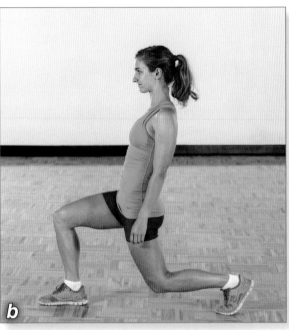

### Execution

1. Start in a lunge position with the left leg back.
2. Slowly lower the back knee toward the floor.
3. Lean the shoulders back and tilt the pelvis forward.
4. Hold for 10 to 30 seconds and repeat 2 or 3 times.
5. Repeat with right leg back.

### MISSTEP
Front knee goes over the toe.

### CORRECTION
Shift your weight until the front knee is over the ankle.

### MISSTEP
Torso leans forward.

### CORRECTION
Keep your back straight and chin parallel to the floor.

## Figure 6.13 **LYING LOW BACK STRETCH**

The low back muscles are used in almost every movement performed, from getting out of bed in the morning to tying your shoes. Prolonged sitting or poor sleeping postures can tighten and stiffen the low back muscles. Tight low back muscles cause pain not only in your low back but also in your hips, pelvis, and legs. Stretching the low back muscles throughout the day helps ease muscle tightness and stiffness. Following is a stretch for the low back.

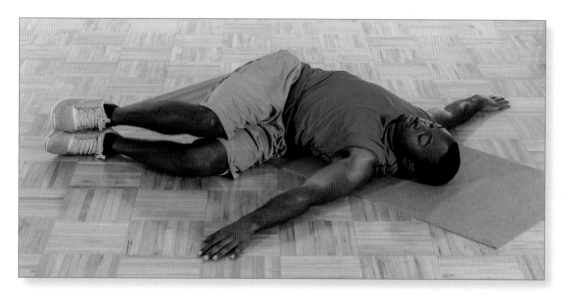

### Execution

1. Lie on back with knees bent.
2. Extend both arms to the sides.
3. Slowly lower both knees to the left.
4. Try to keep the shoulders on the floor.
5. Hold for 10 to 30 seconds and repeat 2 or 3 times.
6. Repeat, lowering the knees to the right.

---

**MISSTEP**

Shoulder comes off the floor.

**CORRECTION**

Shift the knees toward the center until the shoulder rests on the floor.

## Figure 6.14 **LYING ABDOMINAL STRETCH**

Several muscles are in the abdomen; the most prominent is the rectus abdominis. The rectus abdominis can become overstressed by activities you perform every day, such as sitting at a desk for hours or carrying heavy grocery bags. In addition, this muscle assists with breathing. Without full range of motion in the abs, poor posture results and back problems may arise. Following is a stretch for the rectus abdominis.

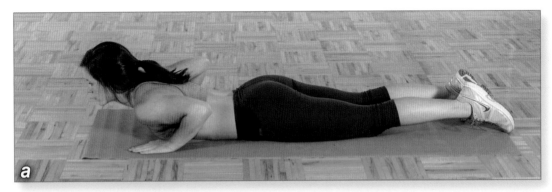

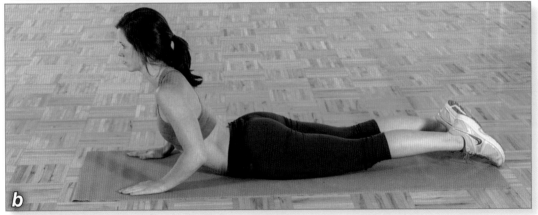

*Execution*

1. Lie flat on the floor with your hands under your shoulders and fingers facing forward.
2. Make sure legs are straight and relax the shoulders back and down.
3. Exhale and slowly lift your chest off the floor, lifting the rib cage but keeping the hips in contact with the floor.
4. Inhale and slowly return to your starting position.

**MISSTEP**

Neck hyperextends.

**CORRECTION**

Keep the eyes focused on the floor between the hands.

**MISSTEP**

Hips rise off the floor.

**CORRECTION**

Bend the arms until the hips lower to the floor.

## Figure 6.15 **OBLIQUE STRETCH**

The obliques (sides of the waist) are used for bending and twisting. Keeping the obliques flexible reduces the chance of a pull, strain, or tear. Following is a stretch for the obliques.

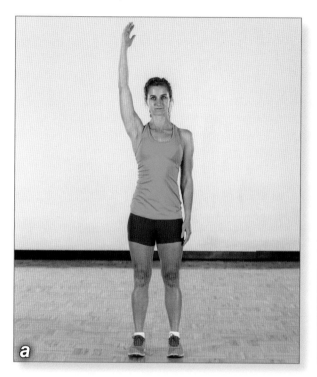

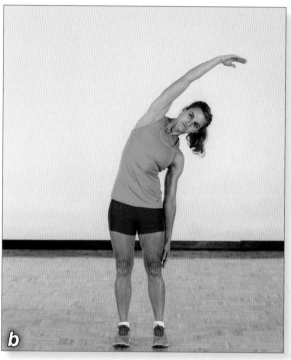

### Execution

1. Stand with feet shoulder-width apart and navel pulled toward the spine.
2. Relax the shoulders back and down, arms by your sides.
3. Reach your right arm up close to your head, keeping the neck neutral.
4. Exhale and slowly reach up and over with your right arm and hold for 10 to 30 seconds.
5. Return to your starting position and repeat on the left side.

### MISSTEP
Hips shift to the side.

### CORRECTION
Keep the legs straight and weight evenly distributed.

### MISSTEP
Torso leans forward.

### CORRECTION
Keep the shoulders, hips, and knees in alignment.

# FLEXIBILITY SUMMARY

Flexibility is an important part of your fitness program, but one of the most neglected. Make sure you take the time to stretch all your major muscles after your workout, especially the areas that are less flexible. And keep in mind that as you age, you become less flexible, which will impact every movement of your body. Remember these exercises can be done most anywhere, and no equipment is needed. You can use this time to rest your mind or as a reward for a job well done!

## Before Taking the Next Step

1. Did you practice the stretches listed in this step? Pay close attention to the areas (if any) that you found to be tight during the assessment in step 1.

2. Did you list the days and times of the week you will be incorporating a stretching routine?

3. Have you practiced slow and controlled breathing?

4. Did you choose a meditation exercise to use in stressful situations?

# Balance

Although you may think of balance training as an issue for older adults, balance training is important for everyone and is a crucial part of fitness. It's in the same group as core strength and flexibility. You need it in order for your body to operate efficiently. Having balance means you are able to maintain your center of gravity over your base of support with minimal postural sway. The base of support is the part of the body that touches the surface supporting you. If you are standing, it's the area between your feet; if you are in a push-up position, it's the area between your hands and feet. You could be an avid runner in great shape but have poor balance. You are not born with balance; you learn it and practice it. It is one of the most neglected areas of fitness.

## FACTORS THAT AFFECT BALANCE

Balance starts to deteriorate as young as age 30 and gets worse with time. You will first notice your lack of balance when you reach for something on the floor and you need to hold on to something for help. Several factors affect balance: vision, kinesthetic awareness, base of support, strength and flexibility, and environment.

### Vision

Vision is a vital part of balance. Your perception changes as your vision changes. When you practice balancing, you retrain the neuromuscular pathways that your brain sends to your working muscles. You are asking these pathways to fire quickly. In turn, this will help you perceive changes in the terrain as you step off a curb, leap over a puddle, or speed up to catch a taxi. In addition, those with vision impairments and those with uncorrected nearsightedness or farsightedness have a greater chance of losing balance.

Inner-ear health is also connected with your balance. The fluid in your inner ear detects your body position. Disorders of the ear such as ear infections, vertigo, and impacted ear wax also affect balance.

### Kinesthetic Awareness

Kinesthetic awareness is how you sense your body. For example, sit in a chair, close your eyes, and raise one arm over your head. How do you know your arm is over your head? You can sense it, or feel it. As the muscles in the shoulder contract, sensors send a message to inform the brain of the change in your position. The position, direction, shape, and effort of your body constantly change, and your kinesthetic awareness detects these changes of body position. You can lower your arm quickly or move it out to the side, and your kinesthetic awareness relays the information to your brain. Balance affects your kinesthetic awareness and vice versa.

## Base of Support

These sensors detect changes in body position with respect to the base of support. When you are standing, your legs are your base of support. When you bring your legs close together, your base of support is narrow and balance is more difficult; when your legs are far apart, the base of support is wide and it is easier to balance. The same is true when sitting: If you sit on a narrow fence dangling your feet, your base of support (fence) makes balancing more difficult than if you were sitting on a sofa with your feet flat on the floor. Your body is constantly balancing throughout the day, adjusting and readjusting as the center of gravity and base of support change.

## Strength and Flexibility

Weak or tight muscles in the legs and hips can affect your balance, and muscle fatigue around the hips and knees affects postural stability. If your muscles are weak you will not be able to balance very long and may have a tendency to lean forward or lean side to side as you walk. If your muscles are tight, you will not have the range of motion some movements may require, which could limit your ability to balance. Climbing stairs is an example in which you must have strong leg and hip muscles to balance on one leg and flexible hip and knee joints to lift your leg up on to the step. You may also have poor balance caused by illness, injury, poor posture, inner-ear problems, or a weak core. More about the core is explained in the following step.

## Environment

Environmental factors, such as surface changes and light conditions, affect balance. For example, it's more difficult to walk on an icy sidewalk or a wet pool deck than on a hardwood floor or concrete sidewalk, and it's easier to walk down a lighted hallway than on one that is dimly lit.

### SUCCESS CHECK

☒ List four factors that may affect your balance.

# BENEFITS OF GOOD BALANCE

Balance training has become more popular recently because it has been recognized as a component of fitness that not only improves quality of life and activities of daily living but your fitness and athletic performance as well. In addition to the physical benefits, there are psychological benefits as well.

Improved balance will aid your fitness routine because balance is the foundation of all movement, whether you are on a treadmill or performing a bench press. As you run, you are balancing each time your foot strikes the ground. When you do a bench press, you are balancing the barbell as well as stabilizing your body on the bench.

If you are already active, balance can reduce injuries. In the past, balance exercises were used mainly in the rehabilitation of injuries, but balance training can also help prevent ankle and knee injuries in recreation and sport. Poor balance is linked to increased risk of ankle injuries and has been found to occur more frequently in men than in women. In addition, balance training helps reduce the recurrence of ankle injuries.

Balance also helps improve spinal stability and posture whether you are immobile or mobile. Examples are when you are sitting at a ball game, standing in line at the movies, climbing stairs, and stepping out of the bathtub.

Older adults benefit from balance exercises—one in three adults suffer from falls each year. Improving your balance can decrease the likelihood of a fall; the strongest predictor of falls is whether or not you have balance. Balance can also help older adults maintain their independence longer by being able to perform activities of daily living without assistance.

Finally, balance exercises help maintain confidence at any age as well as improve self-efficacy (the belief in one's own capabilities). Believing you can complete the exercises in your fitness program helps you to adhere to your plan. The greater your confidence, the better you can perform exercises. This self-confidence can help you take on more difficult tasks and goals.

### SUCCESS CHECK

☒ List at least three benefits of having good balance.

# GUIDELINES AND EQUIPMENT FOR BALANCE

Because balance training is a recent addition to workout programs, there are no specific scientific standards on how often or how long you should practice balance training. The *Physical Activity Guidelines for Americans* (published in 2008 and available at the site www.health.gov/paguidelines/guidelines) state that people should perform balance training at least three times per week. However, you can do balance activities as often as you like, anywhere you like, such as getting up out of a chair without using your hands or balancing on one leg while waiting in line.

The two types of balance are static and dynamic. Static balance is performed while standing still, such as standing on one leg or standing with both feet on a BOSU. Dynamic balance is performed while moving, such as while walking heel to toe or standing on one leg while swinging the other leg or arms. Your balance routine should include both types of balance exercises. The following examples in table 7.1 show how to take a static balance and progress to a dynamic balance.

Although there are specific balance exercises to add to your workout program (see table 7.1), you may also incorporate balancing *as* you perform your workout. This may be helpful if the time you have for exercise is limited. For example, if you usually use a regular stance when performing biceps curls, you can change it to a split stance or try performing a set standing on the right leg and then a set using the left leg.

Table 7.1  Bird Dog Sequence

| Phase | Movement | Difficulty level |
|---|---|---|
| **Step 1**<br>**Start position** | Balance on all fours with hands directly under the shoulders and knees directly under the hips. | **Beginner**<br>Pull the navel toward the spine.<br>Keep spine aligned.<br>Eyes are on the floor.<br> |
| **Step 2**<br>**Static balance** | 1.  Raise one leg off floor.<br>2.  Hold 5 seconds.<br>3.  Repeat with other leg.<br>4.  Raise one arm off floor.<br>5.  Hold 5 seconds.<br>6.  Repeat with other arm.<br>7.  Extend one arm in front and opposite leg behind a few inches off floor.<br>8.  Hold 5 seconds.<br>9.  Repeat on opposite side.<br>10. Extend one arm in front and the opposite leg behind in line with torso.<br>11. Hold 5 seconds.<br>12. Repeat on opposite side. | **Beginner**<br>Start with one leg<br>or one arm at a time.<br><br>**Intermediate**<br>Raise bent arm and<br>leg simultaneously.<br><br>**Advanced**<br>Raise straight arm<br>and leg simultaneously.<br>Increase time.<br> |

| Phase | Movement | Difficulty level |
|-------|----------|------------------|
| Step 3 Dynamic balance | 1. In the static balance position bring your elbow toward your knee under your torso, then back out into extension.<br>2. Do 5 times, then switch to opposite side. | **Intermediate**<br>Use smaller movements and keep arm and leg bent.<br><br><br><br>**Advanced**<br>Use larger movements and extend arm and leg straight. Increase time.<br><br> |
| Step 4 Static balance on ball | 1. Place hips on top of the ball with toes on the floor behind.<br>2. Place hands on floor in front of ball.<br>3. Extend one arm in front and one leg behind until they are in line with torso.<br>4. Hold 5 seconds.<br>5. Repeat on opposite side. | **Intermediate**<br>Place hands and toes farther out from the ball.<br><br><br><br>**Advanced**<br>Place hands and toes close to ball. Increase time.<br><br><br><br>*Make sure size of ball allows hands and toes to touch floor. |

(continued)

**Table 7.1** (continued)

| Step 5 Static balance in push-up position | 1. Place hands and toes in push-up position. 2. Extend one arm and the opposite leg until they are in line with the torso. 3. Hold 5 seconds. 4. Do on opposite side. | Advanced |
|---|---|---|
| Step 6 Dynamic balance in push-up position | 1. Begin in static balance push up position. 2. Extend one arm and opposite leg until they are in line with torso. 3. Simultaneously lower hand and foot until they are near the floor, then return to starting position. 4. Do 5 times, then switch to opposite side. | Very advanced |

## Guidelines

Performing lunges or step-ups, or standing exercises versus sitting exercises, such as the overhead dumbbell shoulder press, will also help balance. Following are basic strategies for a balance program.

- **Seated.** When you begin incorporating balance exercises, start where you feel challenged but safe. Seated balance exercises are a safe and effective way to begin. Use a stable base such as a chair or bench, then progress to a ball.

- **Support.** If you feel unstable on your feet, use support such as a chair or wall. As your balance improves, you can try letting go, but have the support close by for safety. Progress to no support at all.

- **Visual.** Stand with your feet apart and close your eyes. Feel your body sway and how your body corrects your balance. Once you have mastered a balancing pose, you can progress by closing your eyes, which increases the difficulty of the exercise.

- **Focus.** Looking at something stationary (having a focal point) makes it easier to keep your balance. Choose something at a distance, not close by. Progress to moving your focus side to side or up and down.

- **Base of Support.** A wide base of support is the easiest place to start when learning to balance. Progress to narrowing your base of support by putting the feet together, and then try using one leg.

- **Planes of Movement.** Practice balance exercises in all three planes of movement: front to back, side to side, and rotational. Start with short levers (bent arms and legs), then progress to long levers by straightening your arms and legs.

- **Surface.** Start by performing balances on a firm surface. Progress to a soft surface, such as a mat, and then to an inflated surface, such as a balance disc or BOSU.

# Equipment

Many types of balance equipment can improve and challenge your balance exercises:

A **balance disc** (figure 7.1) is a flat, pillow-shaped disc that can be inflated for various levels of balance. The more air in the disc, the more difficult it is to balance.

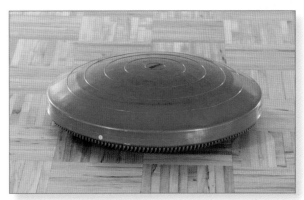

**Figure 7.1** Balance disc.

**Exercise balls** come in various sizes, and ideally you should choose a ball that allows your thighs to be parallel to the floor when sitting (figure 7.2). And, like the balance disc, the more inflated the ball, the more difficult it is to balance. It is versatile with many balance exercises.

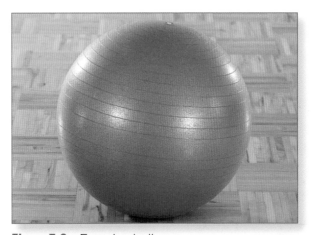

**Figure 7.2** Exercise ball.

**BOSU** stands for *both sides up* because it can be used on either side. This half ball has a flat surface on one side and is inflated on the other (figure 7.3). The rounded side against the floor provides a highly unstable surface, and the flat side down provides an ideal surface for standing exercises.

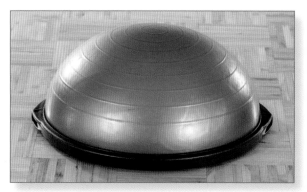

**Figure 7.3**   BOSU ball.

A **Wobble board** may be rounded for a full plane of instability or made to move side to side or forward or backward (figure 7.4). It is made of wood or hard plastic and is highly unstable.

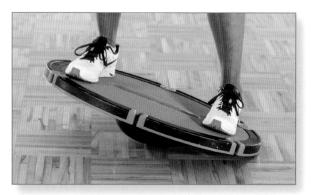

**Figure 7.4**   Wobble board.

**Half or whole foam rollers** (figure 7.5) can be used in a similar way to a balance beam for balance exercises or used with the feet perpendicular to create a more unstable surface.

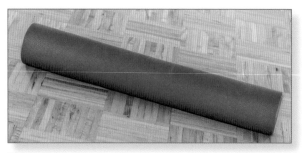

**Figure 7.5**   Foam roller.

Keep in mind that equipment is not necessary for practicing balance exercises—you can work on your balance training by doing some simple yoga poses or tai chi. There are many types of yoga, but you can start with some basic poses such as the tree pose. (Shift your weight to one foot. Bend the knee and draw your foot up to make contact with the inside of the support leg.) Tai chi involves a series of slow, focused movements accompanied by deep breathing. Each posture flows into the next, and your body is in constant motion.

# BALANCE EXERCISES

Figure 7.6 **WEIGHT SHIFT**

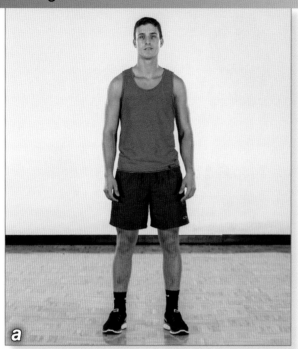
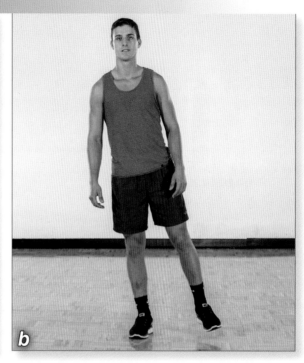

*Preparation*

1. Stand with feet hip-width apart.
2. Pull the navel toward the spine and relax the shoulders back and down.

*Movement*

1. Exhale and slowly lean to the right, shifting your body weight to the right foot.

2. Allow the left foot to rise off the floor to the side of the body.
3. Hold 5 seconds (about 2 long, deep breaths).
4. Inhale and slowly return to the starting position.
5. Repeat leaning to the left side, shifting body weight to the left foot.

**Progression 1**

Increase to 10 seconds (about 4 long, deep breaths).

**Progression 2**

Perform with eyes closed.

---

**MISSTEP**

Torso leans forward.

**CORRECTION**

Keep the shoulders, hips, and knees in alignment.

**MISSTEP**

Head and neck pull forward.

**CORRECTION**

Keep chin parallel to the floor.

Figure 7.7    **FOAM ROLLER BALANCE**

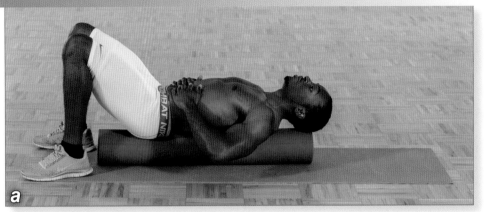

### Preparation

1.  Lie on your back with your head, spine, and hips in contact with the foam roller.
2.  Place your feet shoulder-width apart and hands on your abdomen.
3.  Pull your navel toward the spine and relax your shoulders down and back.

### Movement

1.  Move the feet together and hold for 10 to 30 seconds.

### Progression 1

1.  Extend the right arm up and the left arm down so they are parallel to the floor.
2.  Alternate arms for 10 to 30 seconds.

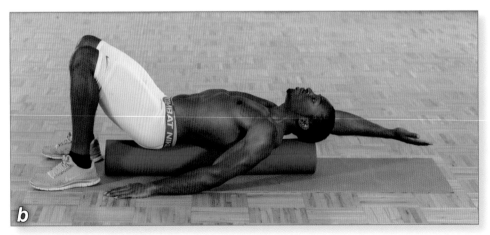

Progression 1

**Progression 2**

1. With arms straight but not locked, hold a medicine ball over the chest.
2. Lower behind the head until the arms are parallel to the floor.
3. Return to the starting position.
4. Do for 10 to 30 seconds.

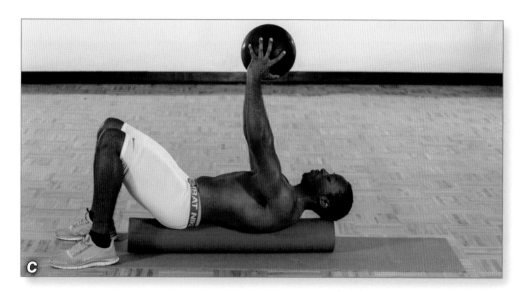

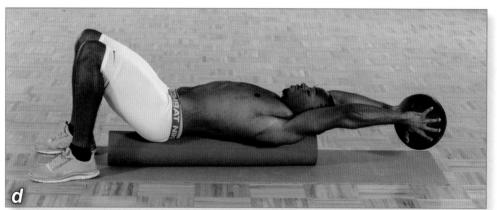

Progression 2

*(continued)*

**Figure 7.7** *(continued)*

**Progression 3**

1. With arms straight but not locked, hold a medicine ball over the chest.
2. Lower to the left side until the arms are at the 10 o'clock position.
3. Return to the starting position.
4. Repeat to the right side.
5. Do for 10 to 30 seconds.

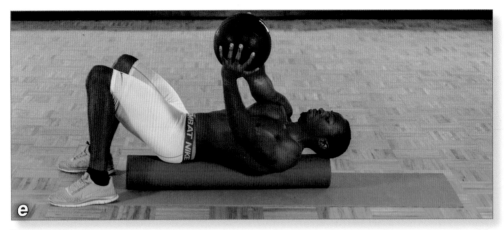

Progression 3

**Progression 4**

1. With hands on abdomen, extend the left leg until the knees are even.
2. Hold for 10 to 30 seconds.
3. Repeat, raising the right leg.

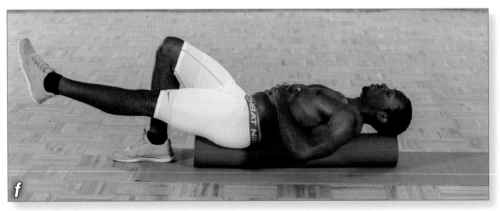

Progression 4

**MISSTEP**

You cannot maintain balance.

**CORRECTION**

Place feet farther apart.

## Figure 7.8  ONE-LEG BALANCE

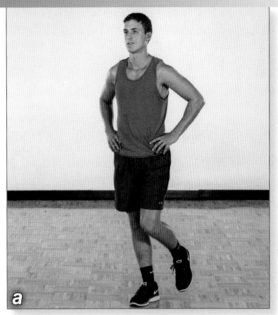

### Preparation

1. Stand with the feet shoulder-width apart and pull the navel toward the spine.
2. Relax the shoulders back and down, and place your hands on your hips.

### Movement

1. Shift your weight to the right leg and slowly bend the left knee, lifting the foot off the floor.
2. Hold for up to 30 seconds, then repeat with your weight on the left leg.

### Progression 1

1. Swing the leg forward about 45 degrees, then behind about 45 degrees.
2. Do 8 to 10 times.

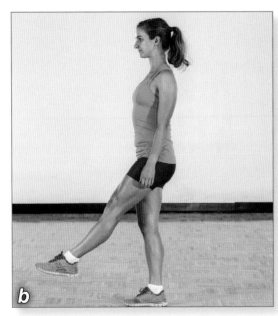
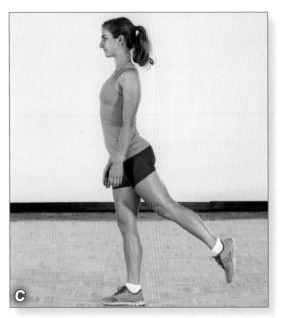

Progression 1

*(continued)*

**Figure 7.8** *(continued)*

**Progression 2**

Place a cone near the support leg and reach the opposite arm downward to touch the cone.

**Progression 3**

Use a BOSU or balance disc to balance on one leg.

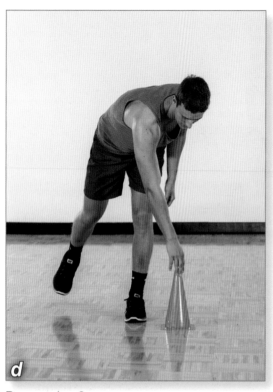

Progression 2

Progression 3

---

### MISSTEP
Torso leans forward.

### CORRECTION
Keep back straight and chin parallel to the floor.

### MISSTEP
You place the raised foot against the standing leg.

### CORRECTION
Keep the elevated foot in the air.

Figure 7.9 **SINGLE-LEG BALANCE WITH TORSO ROTATION**

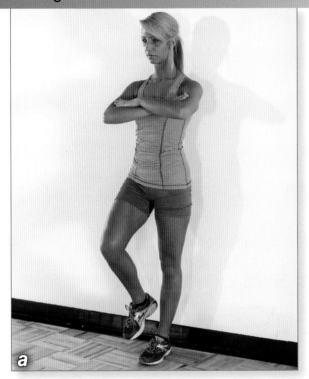 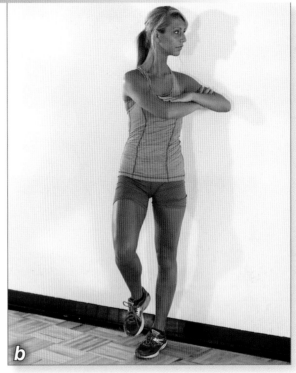

*Preparation*

1. Stand on your left leg 6 inches (15 cm) from a wall and cross the arms over the chest.
2. Pull the navel toward your spine and relax the shoulders back and down.

**Progression 1**

Touch the shoulder to the wall.

**Progression 2**

Repeat for 45 seconds.

*Movement*

1. Exhale and slowly turn the torso to the left, keeping the hips and toes of the support leg facing front.
2. Inhale and slowly return to the starting position.
3. Hold for 30 seconds, then repeat using the left leg.

**MISSTEP**

Torso leans forward.

**CORRECTION**

Keep back straight and chin parallel to the floor.

## Figure 7.10 **BALL SIT BALANCE**

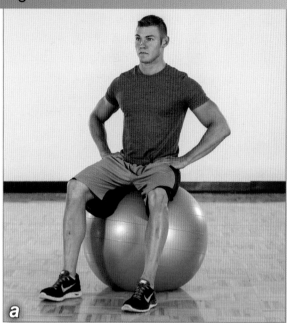

### Preparation

1. Sit on the top of the exercise ball with both feet securely on the floor shoulder-width apart.
2. Keep your back straight and place your hands on your hips.
3. Pull the navel toward the spine and relax your shoulders back and down.

### Progression 1

1. Narrow the base of support by moving the feet together.
2. Hold for 5 to 10 seconds.

### Progression 2

1. Slowly lift your right foot off the floor.
2. Hold for 5 to 10 seconds.
3. Return the right foot to the floor and repeat with the left foot.
4. Hold for 5 to 10 seconds.

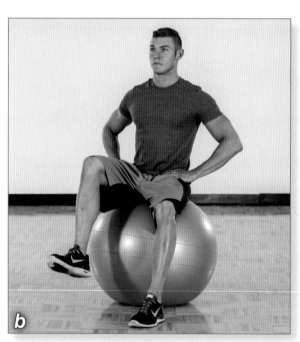

Progression 2

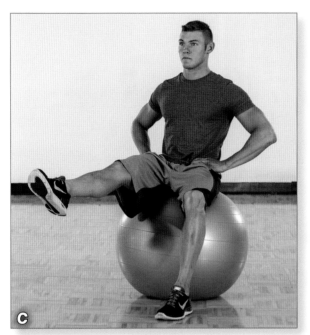

Progression 3

### Progression 3

1. Slowly lift your right leg straight out in front.
2. Hold for 5 to 10 seconds.
3. Return the right foot to the floor and repeat with the left foot.
4. Hold for 5 to 10 seconds.

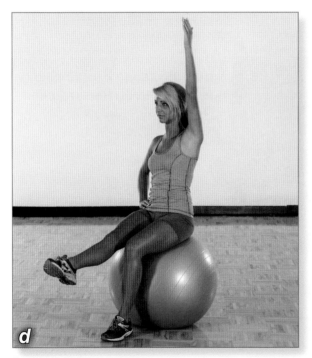

Progression 4

### Progression 4

Add arm movements up and down while holding the leg off the floor.

**MISSTEP**

Upper back rounds.

**CORRECTION**

Keep your back straight and chin parallel to the floor.

**MISSTEP**

You move too much in trying to balance.

**CORRECTION**

Place the feet farther apart.

Figure 7.11 **STANDING TOE TAP**

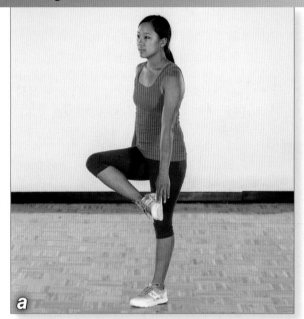
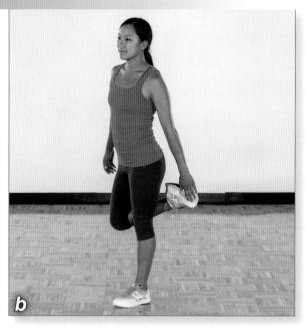

**Preparation**

1. Stand on the left leg.
2. Pull the navel toward your spine and relax the shoulders down and back.

**Movement**

1. Exhale and slowly touch the left hand to the right foot in front of the torso.
2. Inhale and slowly return to the starting position.
3. Exhale and slowly touch the left hand to the right foot behind the torso.

4. Inhale and slowly return to the starting position.
5. Do for 30 seconds.
6. Repeat the sequence standing on the right leg using the right hand to the left foot.

**Progression 1**

Increase time to 45 seconds.

**Progression 2**

Increase time to 60 seconds.

**MISSTEP**

Torso bends too far forward.

**CORRECTION**

Lift the leg higher to meet the hand.

Figure 7.12  **BOSU SQUAT**

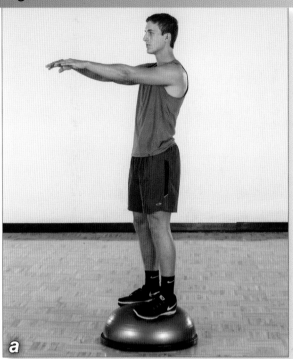

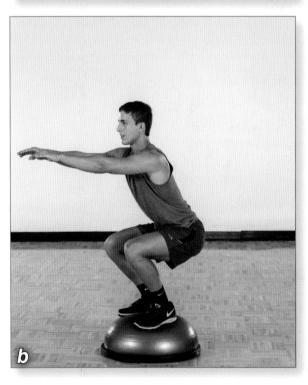

*Preparation*

1. Stand with feet shoulder-width apart and pull navel toward the spine.
2. Relax the shoulders back and down.

*Movement*

1. Exhale and slowly lower the hips, keeping the back straight. Move the arms forward until they are parallel to the floor as you squat.
2. Inhale and slowly return to the starting position.
3. Perform 5 to 8 reps.

*(continued)*

**Figure 7.12** *(continued)*

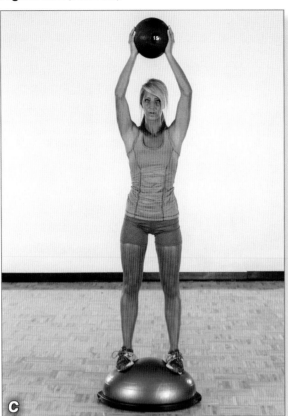

## Progression 1

Add a medicine ball movement or reverse the BOSU.

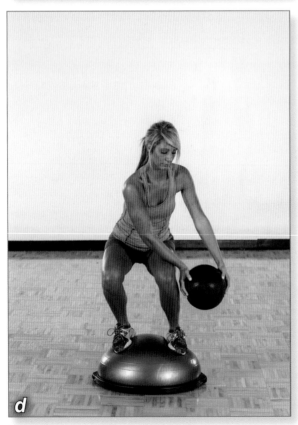

Progression 1: Ball movement.

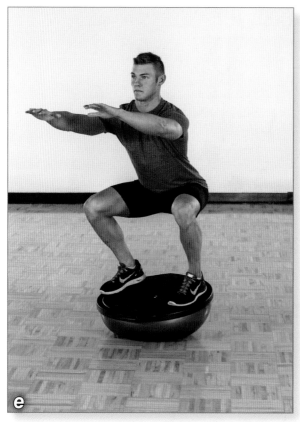

Progression 1: Reverse the BOSU.

### MISSTEP
Upper body leans forward.

### CORRECTION
Straighten the back and keep the chin parallel to the floor.

### MISSTEP
Movement in the hips and legs is not simultaneous.

### CORRECTION
Bend the knees and lower the hips at the same time.

Figure 7.13 **STANDING REACH**

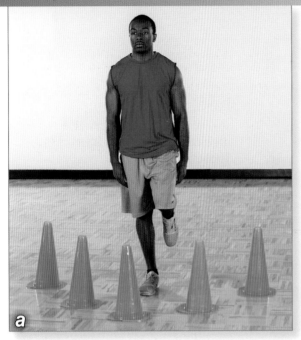

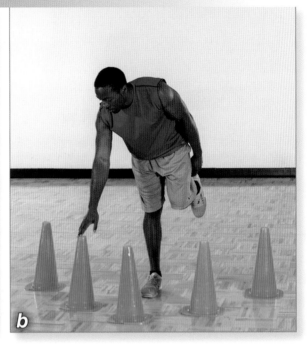

*Preparation*

1. Place 3 to 5 small cones (you can use soup cans) within reach at 10 o'clock, 11 o'clock, 12 o'clock, 1 o'clock, and 2 o'clock positions.
2. Stand on the right leg behind the middle cone.
3. Pull the navel toward your spine.

*Movement*

1. Inhale slowly; with the right hand, touch farthest cone on the left side.
2. Exhale and slowly return to the starting position.

3. Repeat, touching each cone with the right hand.
4. Repeat the sequence standing on the right leg and using the left hand.

**Progression 1**

1. Use 3 cones at 11 o'clock, 12 o'clock, and 1 o'clock.
2. Increase speed.

**Progression 2**

1. Add cones at 10 o'clock and 2 o'clock.
2. Increase speed.

## Figure 7.14  STAR BALANCE

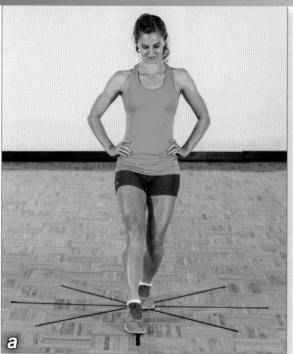

### Preparation

1. Place 4 pieces of tape evenly on the floor into an 8-point star.

2. Stand in the center and balance on your left leg, navel toward the spine. Relax the shoulders back and down. Your right foot is the tapper.

### Movement

1. Reach your right foot toward the front tape as far as you can and tap the floor, then return to center, maintaining your balance on the left leg.

2. Repeat, reaching your right foot to the next strip of tape in a clockwise direction, then return to center.

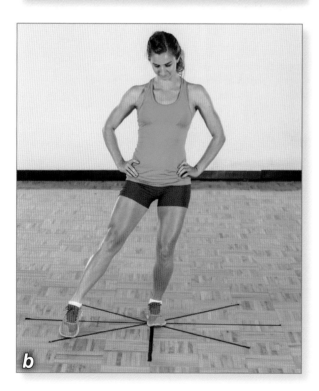

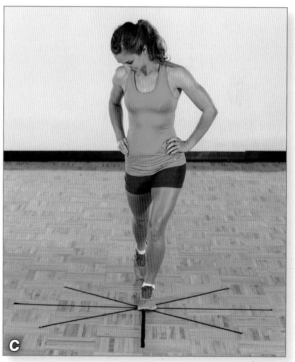

*(continued)*

**Figure 7.14** *(continued)*

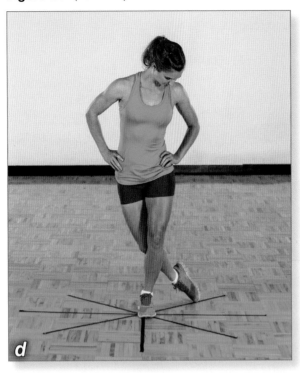

3. Continue until you have tapped all 8 strips of tape.

4. Repeat with your weight on your right leg, using the left foot as the tapper and going in a clockwise direction.

5. Make sure your knee doesn't rotate; keep it facing forward.

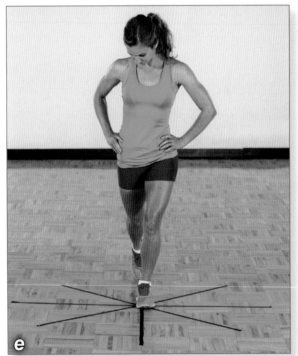

**Figure 7.14** Star balance.

### MISSTEP
Supporting leg rotates.

### CORRECTION
Keep the support leg (knee) facing forward.

**MISSTEP**

Upper body leans forward.

**CORRECTION**

Keep your back straight and chin parallel to the floor.

Although you may have time in your schedule to perform 15 to 20 minutes 3 times a week for balance exercises, you may not have extra time to dedicate to balance. However, you can incorporate balance without adding extra time to your workout plan. You can use balance exercises as a warm-up before exercising, or you can use balance exercises as a cool-down at the end. You can also perform balance exercises during weight training exercises.

As a warm-up or cool-down, you can perform 3 to 4 minutes of walking on a beam or complete the star balance sequence. For example, start the sequence of the star balance by first reaching your foot halfway way toward the line. For the second round, reach your foot three quarters toward the line, and reach your foot to the end of the line on the third round. A beginner can do the star balance using just 4 lines instead of 8 (which are shorter in length).

# ONE-LEG BALANCE WARM-UP OR COOL-DOWN SEQUENCE

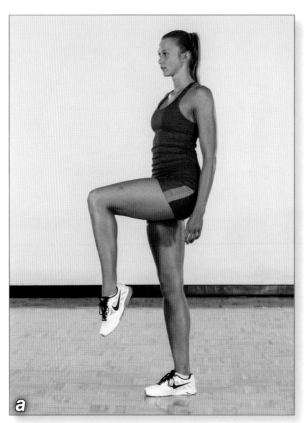

1. Static one-leg balance
2. Leg swing front to back
3. Side leg swing
4. Leg circle

Start with a static balance on one foot for 10 seconds (figure 7.15a), then add movement (dynamic balance): Swing the leg forward and back for 10 reps (b and c) and then out to the side for 10 reps (d). Add foot circles, completing 10 clockwise and 10 counterclockwise (e). Beginners can perform 5 reps each or stand close to a wall if support is needed, and advanced exercisers can perform the balance sequence on the BOSU or balance disc (see figure 7.16).

**Figure 7.15** One leg balance warm-up or cool-down.

*(continued)*

**Figure 7.15** *(continued)*

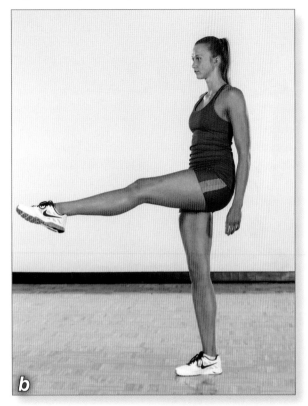

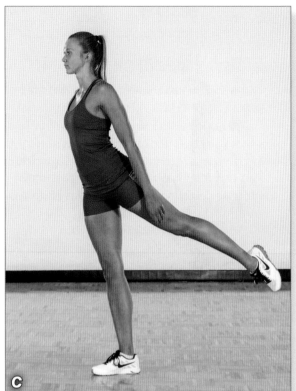

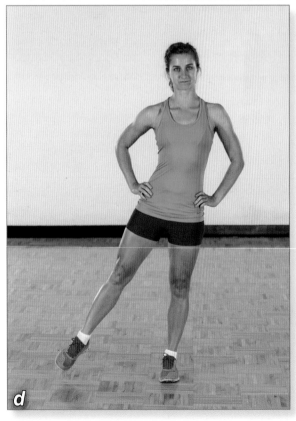

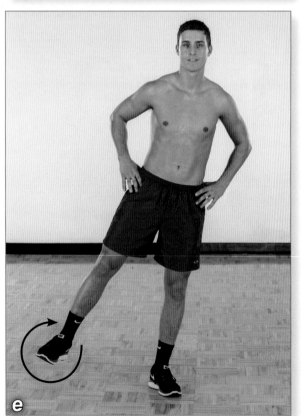

During your workout, you can exchange many of the exercises that are usually done standing on two feet with standing on one foot, such as standing dumbbell or barbell curl or an overhead dumbbell shoulder press. If you currently perform 3 sets of biceps curls, begin by performing 1 set balancing on the right leg and 1 set balancing on the left leg (figure 7.17a). Once the exercise becomes easy on one leg, you can try using a BOSU dome-side up (figure 7.17b); for more advanced exercise, do it dome-side down (figure 7.17c).

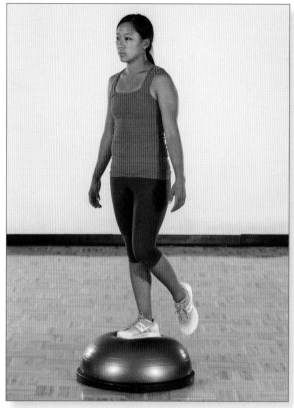

**Figure 7.16**   One-leg balance using BOSU.

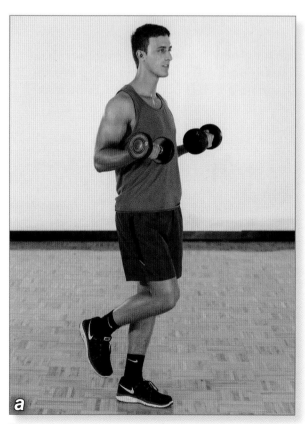

**Figure 7.17a**   One-leg balance using dumbbells.

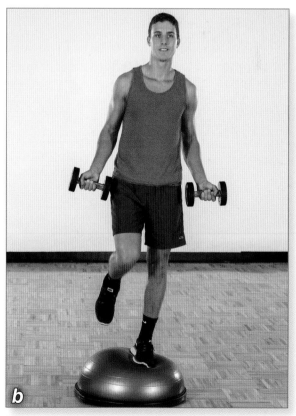

**Figure 7.17b**   One-leg balance using dumbbells and BOSU.

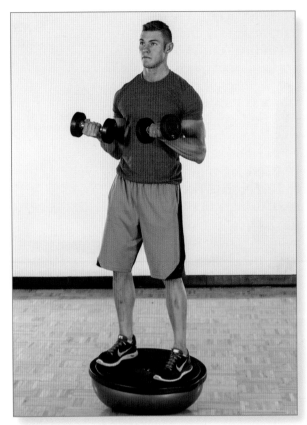

**Figure 7.17c**   One-leg balance using dumbbells and reverse BOSU.

The stability ball or BOSU can be substituted for a bench or a seat in exercises that require you to sit or lie either on your back or front (figure 7.18). Or you can also perform body-weight exercises such as the squat or push-up on a BOSU (figure 7.19). Start with performing 1 set of your exercise on the BOSU or ball, then increase to 2 sets or more.

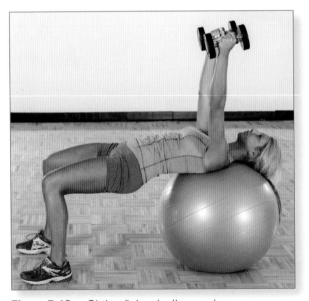

**Figure 7.18**   Sitting/lying ball exercises.

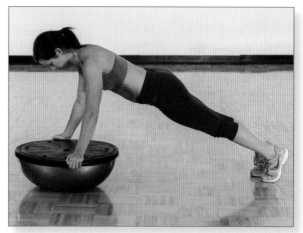

**Figure 7.19** Body-weight exercises using reverse BOSU.

Another option to add balance to your fitness program is to take an exercise from your current fitness program (such as the push-up) and for 2 weeks use the BOSU. After 2 weeks, change to a different exercise (triceps) and use the exercise ball for seated overhead extension (figure 7.20). After 2 weeks, change to another exercise and add balance, and so on.

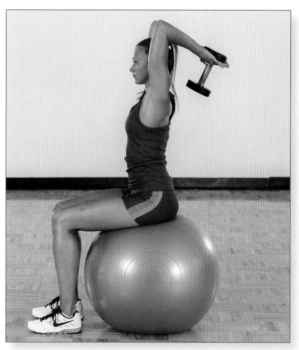

**Figure 7.20** Seated overhead triceps extension.

### SUCCESS CHECK

☒ Choose a balance exercise that suits your fitness level.

☒ List at least two progressions for the balance exercise that would be more challenging.

# BALANCE SUMMARY

Balance is an important part of fitness because it affects your everyday life from the time you get out of bed until you crawl back into bed at the end of the day. Remember that if you don't have the time to perform individual routines for balance, you can incorporate balance into your workout or throughout the day (standing on one leg while doing dishes or washing your hands).

## Before Taking the Next Step

1. Did you choose one or two balances to add to your fitness program?

2. Do you have access to any equipment needed for your balance exercises?

3. Did you list the days and times of the week you will be incorporating balance into your fitness routine?

# Core Strength and Stability

The core, sometimes referred to as the powerhouse, can be described as the link between the upper and lower body. Many people concentrate on the outer abdominal muscles that make up a six-pack because they are visible, and mistakenly call this their core. Because most core muscles are not visible, they tend to be neglected, but they are vital to overall health, fitness, and athletic performance. The core consists of all the muscles from the rib cage to the pelvis, including those that wrap around the spinal column and surround the vital organs.

The core stabilizes the normal S-curve of the spine in spite of the activity that is being performed, whether it is sitting, performing a squat, or hitting a tennis ball. These muscles shift the body weight, transfer energy, and help control movement. All movement either originates in the core or moves through the core from the upper body to the lower body and vice versa.

The normal S-curve as shown in figure 8.1 is the natural position of the spinal column when viewed from the side. The pressure that is put on the spine is distributed more evenly with a normal S-shaped spinal column. That is why it is so important to maintain a neutral spine (navel toward the spine and shoulders relaxed back and down) when performing basic movements such as squat, push-up, biceps curl, walking, and sitting.

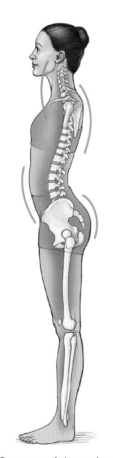

**Figure 8.1**   S-curve of the spine.

# MUSCLES OF THE CORE

We will identify six main muscle groups, their locations, and their purpose. Keep in mind that these muscles either stabilize the core or provide movement in the core.

## Rectus Abdominis

One of the most well-known muscles is the rectus abdominis—the muscles that create the six-pack and can be seen in figure 8.2. These two thin, long muscles run vertically down the front of the body and are attached from the sternum to the pelvis. They are horizontally connected by fibrous bands (not attachments). These muscles allow the body to bend forward and stabilize the upper body when you are carrying a heavy load. The rectus abdominis also helps with breathing when exhaling forcefully.

## Obliques

The external obliques are the largest abdominal muscles that run diagonally downward and inward on the front of the body, forming a V-shape (see figure 8.3). They move the torso side to side. The internal obliques lie under the external obliques and wrap around the spine to the middle of the abdomen. They allow the body to bend and rotate to the side as well as support the spine during movement. They are known as the same-side rotators because they act in opposition of the external obliques. For example, if you are turning to the right, the right internal obliques and the left external obliques are engaged.

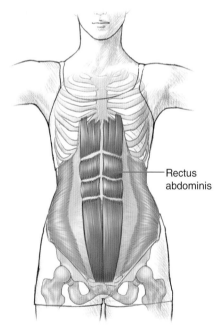

**Figure 8.2**  Rectus abdominis.

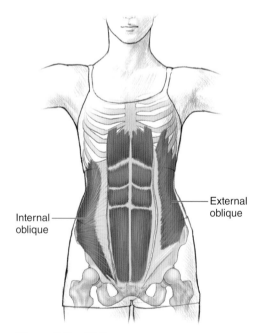

**Figure 8.3**  Obliques.

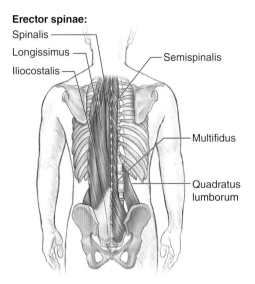

Erector spinae:
Spinalis
Longissimus
Iliocostalis
Semispinalis
Multifidus
Quadratus lumborum

**Figure 8.4** Erector spinae.

## Erector Spinae

The erector spinae muscles are actually a group of muscles that run along the spine (see figure 8.4) and work with the abdominal muscles to support the upper body and keep the spine erect whether you are sitting, running, or standing at the sink doing dishes. These neglected but important set of core muscles also move the body side to side and are crucial for good posture.

## Transversus Abdominis

The transversus abdominis is a deeper layer of abdominal muscles shown in figure 8.5. These muscles stabilize the low back, especially during movement. They also surround and help protect the internal organs. Notice this is the mus cle you brace when someone is about to hit you in the abdomen! The muscles wrap horizontally around the torso similar to a corset. The multifidi muscles act as the laces in that corset (transversus abdominis). They are the smallest but most powerful muscles that support the spine. They help take the pressure off the spinal discs by distributing weight along the S-curve of the spine. They are also the first muscles to be activated and recruited before an actual movement, such as opening a car door or performing a lunge.

## Pelvic Floor

The pelvic floor lies under the pelvis and acts as a hammock or minitrampoline that supports the bladder and other organs. It is important for both men and women to have strong pelvic floor muscles because they support the bladder and bowel. The pelvic floor should be engaged in all exercises.

Multifidus

Transverse abdominals (TVA)

Pelvic floor

**Figure 8.5** Transversus abdominis.

## Diaphragm

The diaphragm is a dome-shaped core muscle that separates the chest from the abdominal cavity and is the main respiratory muscle as shown in figure 8.6. When you inhale, the diaphragm contracts and makes the chest cavity expand, causing a suction that brings air into the lungs. This reduces intrathoracic pressure and is why proper breathing during exercise is crucial. Always exhale during the exertion of an exercise—when the movement of the exercise is most difficult, such as the up phase of a biceps curl or the up phase of a push-up.

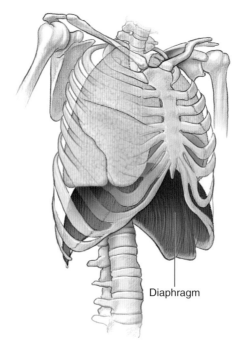

Diaphragm

**Figure 8.6**  Diaphragm.

# FACTORS THAT AFFECT THE CORE

Factors that affect the core include your occupation, activities and sports, prolonged sitting, and general fitness. Many jobs require a lot of bending forward, such as construction, plumbing, and restocking shelves, which affect posture. Your job might entail carrying a load on one side, such as delivering mail or holding a baby on the hip. These positions cause posture abnormalities.

Many people spend hours in a seated position at computers or desks. But whether you are sitting at a job, watching TV, riding in a car, or eating dinner, prolonged sitting can have a harmful effect. Your abdominal muscles become shortened and erector spinae muscles become elongated and weak. Over time this muscle imbalance can cause hyperkyphosis, a forward curving posture that is characteristic of your seated prolonged posture. Take a break from prolonged sitting, or use an exercise ball instead of a chair. When using an exercise ball, the tiny movements created by maintaining stability cause the core muscles to be engaged. When sitting, follow these guidelines to ensure you have proper form:

- Sit upright and relax your shoulders back and down.
- Keep the back of your pelvis against the back of the seat to prevent slouching.
- Use a lumbar support or small pillow to support the natural curve in your low back.
- Chair height should accommodate feet flat on the floor with a 90-degree bend at the knee (use a small footrest if your chair is too high).
- Try not to cross your legs, because that rotates the pelvis backward and raises one hip, which puts pressure on the other hip and results in your back being out of alignment.
- Keep elbows bent 90 degrees and close to the body.
- Keep hands, wrists, and forearms parallel to the floor.
- Make sure the top of your computer monitor is at about eye level.
- Stand and stretch 1 minute for every 20 to 30 minutes of sitting.

Another factor that affects your core is activities and sports. Although being active and participating in sports are undeniably encouraged, some can have an adverse effect on your core. For example, riding for hours on a racing bicycle where your upper body is slung low over the handlebars can cause core back muscles to be overstretched and abdominal muscles to be tight. Those who run for hours every day may develop a forward head position and forward body lean, which may affect posture muscles along the spine. Poor posture muscles of the spine and pelvis can cause low back pain.

The last factor that affects the core is your general fitness. Muscles must be both strong and flexible. Core muscles must be strong to support the spine and support the movement of your upper and lower body, but if the opposing core muscles are tight, it becomes difficult to maintain that support. For example, you may have very strong low back muscles and weak abdominals, and this imbalance can lead to fatigue, pain, and injury. On the other hand, overtraining ab muscles and getting a rippling six-pack while ignoring low back muscles can set you up for low back pain and injuries.

### SUCCESS CHECK

- ☒ List four factors that may affect your core.
- ☒ What muscles are involved in the core?
- ☒ What is an S-curve?

# BENEFITS OF A STRONG CORE

A strong core enhances balance, stability, recreational activities and sports, your job, and activities of daily living. It helps you maintain a healthy back, improves posture, and reduces the risk of injuries.

A strong core and balance go hand in hand. Research has shown that as core strength increases, balance improves. Better balance and stability due to a strong core can reduce your risk of injuries from falling. In addition, a strong core will stabilize your body no matter what direction you are moving, whether it is getting up from an office chair or performing walking lunges.

No matter where the movement begins in sport or recreational activities, it transfers either from the core or up and down through the core. You may think that when you move, your arms and legs do most of the work. On the contrary—the movement starts at the core and moves outward. How well your upper body or lower body functions is directly related to the strength of your core. This will certainly affect activities such as in-line skating, doing a yoga pose, and returning a tennis serve.

Your job can benefit from having a strong core, whether you are a construction worker lifting and twisting or an office worker. Sitting at a desk demands a strong core as well. A strong core helps you engage in good posture, which can keep muscles from becoming fatigued on the job. This is also true when you are performing activities of daily living such as lifting, carrying, reaching, mopping, and bending. All these activities originate from the core.

About 20 percent of people will suffer at some point from low back pain or low back injuries. A weak core does not provide adequate spine support and may put you at risk for a herniated disc. Core exercises are often prescribed to alleviate low back pain and prevent the injury from reoccurring. Weak core muscles can lead to slouching, which not only increases wear and tear on your spine but also makes breathing deeply more difficult. A strong core supports good posture because it makes you stand taller with your limbs in alignment. Good posture lengthens the spine and allows it full range of motion in flexing and extending. Good posture also opens up the airway, making it easier to inhale and exhale, and it makes you look and feel better.

A strong core ensures all the systems in the torso not only are protected but can also go about performing their work as you move your body throughout the day. These systems are the internal organs, central nervous system, and some of the body's principal veins and arteries. If you have persistent pressure on part of your spine due to weak core muscles, it will sooner or later affect your movement and cause pain.

Upright posture caused by a strong core can help with self-confidence. A person standing tall gives the impression of being confident and in control of her life, whereas a person who slouches can give the impression of being weak and defeated. A strong core provides you with better control of your muscles and takes some of the strain from other muscle groups that may be overworked.

### SUCCESS CHECK

☒  List at least three benefits of having a strong core.

# CORE EXERCISES

Working the core is not just performing several rounds of crunches to failure but working all the muscle groups involved from the rib cage to the pelvis. The five components of core stability are motor control, function, strength, endurance, and flexibility. No matter how strong you are or how much endurance you have, without motor control and function in the core, the other three components are ineffective.

You must have core stability to support and protect the spine. The better your core stability, the lower the risk of injury. First find your neutral spine by performing the cat–cow exercise (figure 8.7).

## Figure 8.7 **CAT–COW**

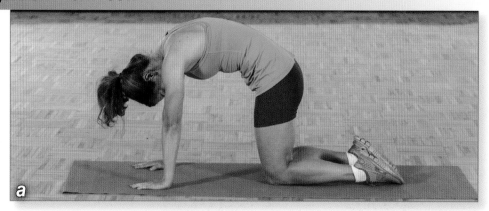

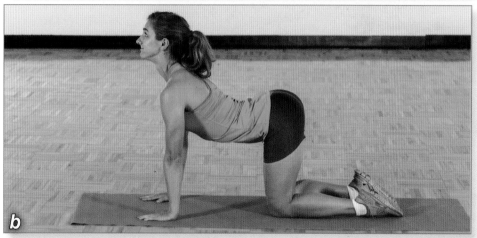

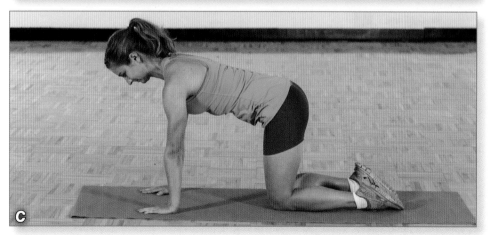

### Preparation

1. Get on all fours (knees directly under the hips and hands directly under the shoulders).

### Movement

1. Round your back into a cat stretch
2. Arch your back into a cow posture.

3. Finally, position your spine halfway between cat and cow. This is neutral spine.

4. Your gaze is toward the floor; the back of your head, shoulder blades, and low back are in a straight line.

Once you are able to activate a neutral spine on hands and knees, try keeping a neutral spine in a plank position (shown in figure 8.8) and then a push-up position, keeping the head, shoulder blades, and low back aligned. Practice each of these stabilization positions until you can hold them for 60 seconds.

**Figure 8.8   PLANK**

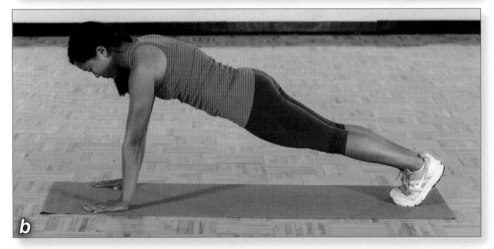

**Figure 8.8**   Proper plank position on elbows (*a*) with straightened arms (*b*). Improper position on elbows or arms (*c*).

## Figure 8.9  BIRD DOG

Progress to movement while maintaining core stability. This mobility sequence starts on all fours with a neutral spine. Slowly lift the left arm parallel to the floor, keeping the core stable (not moving). Repeat with the right arm and then left leg and right leg. Hold for 2 to 5 rounds of deep breathing. To make sure your core is stable, place a foam roller across your low back and repeat the exercises. The foam roller should remain level at all times. If you are moving your spine, you do not have core stability.

**All-Fours**

Keep a long neck, and keep your shoulders away from your ears (a).

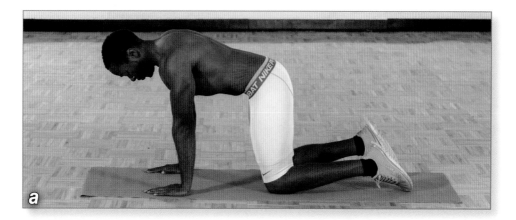

**One Arm**

- Extend (not raise) the arm parallel to the floor (b).
- Don't let the chest sink or the shoulder blades roll inward.
- Alternate left arm and right arm for 2 sets of 5 reps each.

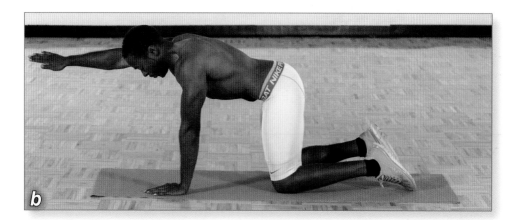

*(continued)*

**Figure 8.9** *(continued)*

**One Leg**

- Extend (not raise) the leg *(c)*.
- The stable spine should be in a neutral (slightly arched) position) and ab muscles engaged.
- Alternate left leg and right leg for 2 sets of 5 reps each.

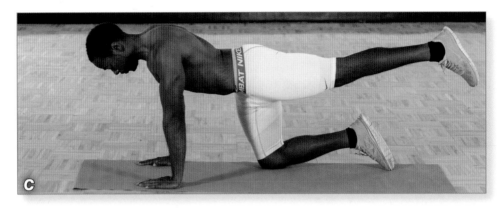

**Foam Roller (or medicine ball)**

- Check your core stability during these exercises with a foam roller or medicine ball placed on the low back *(d)*.
- Keep the foam roller (or medicine ball) stable.
- Progress to the next step of moving your left arm and right leg simultaneously, keeping a neutral spine and core stability *(e)*.
- Repeating the movement on one side trains endurance; alternating sides trains movement initiation.

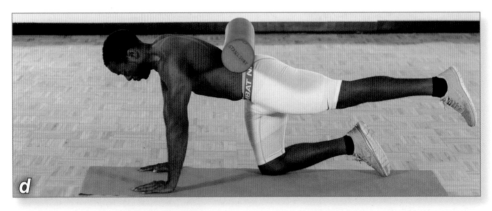

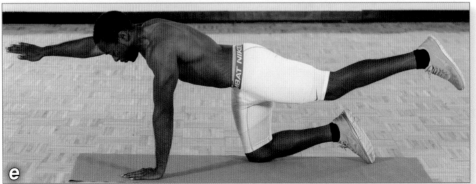

**Sample Progressions**

*2 sets of 5 reps each*

*Make sure you breathe—do not hold your breath.*

### Progression 1

1. In bird dog position, lower the arm and leg simultaneously to the floor, then back to the starting position (*f*).
2. Use the foam roller to ensure core stability.

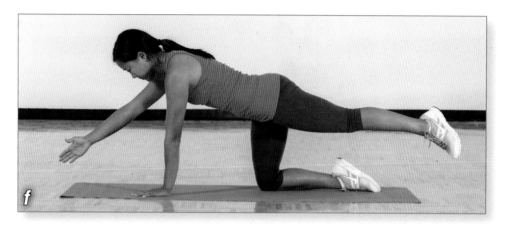

### Progression 2

1. In bird dog position, circle the arm and leg simultaneously clockwise, then counterclockwise (*g* ).
2. Make sure the movement comes from the shoulder and hip.
3. Use the foam roller to ensure core stability.

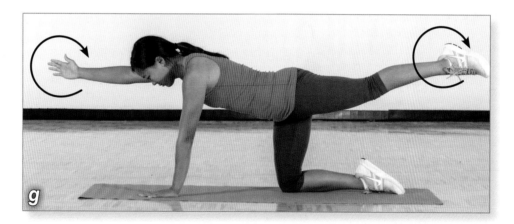

*(continued)*

**Figure 8.9** *(continued)*

*Progression 3*

1. In bird dog position, bring the elbow toward the knee, then extend (*h*).
2. Use the foam roller to ensure core stability because your back may tend to arch beyond neutral.

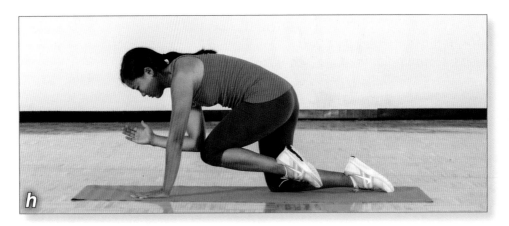

### MISSTEP
Low back moves.

### CORRECTION
Contract the abdominals throughout the movement.

### MISSTEP
Momentum lifts the leg and arm up.

### CORRECTION
Think about extending the leg and the arm instead of lifting.

### MISSTEP
Head and neck pull down.

### CORRECTION
Focus eyes directly on the floor and keep the back of the head in alignment with the upper back.

## Figure 8.10  PELVIC FLOOR CONTRACTION

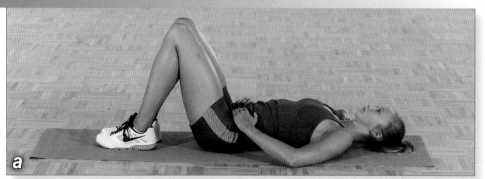

### Preparation

1. Lie on your back with knees bent and feet flat on the floor.
2. Place fingertips 1 inch (2.5 cm) down and 1 inch in from your hip bones as a cue to keep other muscles from contracting (there should be no movement in the abs, butt, or legs).

### Movement

1. Exhale and contract the muscles you would use to stop the flow of urine and hold for 5 to 8 seconds. Feel your pelvic floor lift inward.
2. Inhale and relax.
3. Make sure you are not bearing down, which pushes the pelvic floor down instead of up.
4. Perform 10 to 30 reps 3 to 5 times per week.

### Progression

1. Activate the pelvic floor muscles.
2. Exhale and slowly slide your left heel out, keeping the pelvic floor engaged.
3. Inhale and return to the starting position.
4. Repeat with the right leg.
5. Perform 10 to 30 reps 3 times per week.

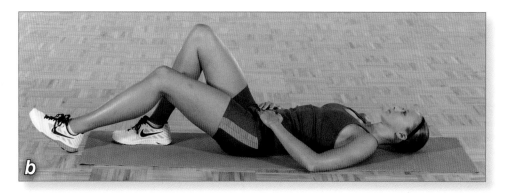

### MISSTEP
Head lifts off the floor.

### CORRECTION
Relax the head and neck onto the floor.

Figure 8.11 **PELVIC TILT**

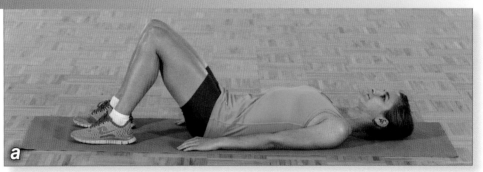

**Preparation**

1. Lie on your back with knees bent and feet flat on the floor.

**Movement**

1. Exhale and slowly contract the pelvic floor, tilt the pelvis back, and slowly roll up onto your shoulders.
2. Inhale and return to the starting position.
3. Perform 10 to 30 reps 3 times per week.

**Progression**

1. Activate the pelvic floor muscles.
2. Exhale and slowly contract the pelvic floor, tilt the pelvis back, and slowly roll up onto your shoulders.
3. In pelvic tilt position lift the right and then left leg as in marching, inhaling and exhaling as you march.
4. Perform 10 to 30 reps 3 times per week.

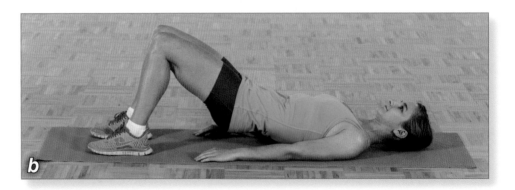

**MISSTEP**

Buttocks lift too high.

**CORRECTION**

Relax the lower back and glutes.

Besides these exercises that isolate specific core muscles, countless activities can strengthen the core. Think about engaging the core while performing functional movements such as deadlift, overhead squat, and push-up and other activities such as boxing, running, and swimming. This involves engaging the pelvic floor, pulling the navel toward the spine, and bracing the abdominal muscles. By doing so, you will acquire more efficient movement and strength.

# SAMPLE CORE STABILITY AND MOBILITY PROGRESSIONS

Add a second set when the movement becomes easy (see workout tables 8.1a and 8.1b).

Table 8.1a    Workout 1: Bird Dog

| Sets and reps | Exercise |
| --- | --- |
| 1 x 5 | Alternate right and left arms |
| 1 x 5 | Alternate right and left legs |
| 1 x 5 | Alternate right arm and left leg, left arm and right leg |

Table 8.1b    Workout 2: Bird Dog

| Sets and reps | Exercise |
| --- | --- |
| 1 x 10 | Alternate right and left legs |
| 1 x 10 | Alternate right arm and left leg, left arm and right leg |
| 1 x 10 | Alternate right and left arms |
| 1 x 10 | Alternate right arm and left leg, left arm and right leg |

Depending on how well you are able to stabilize the core, you should perform these exercises at least a few times a week. Once you have developed your core stability, you can progress to the more superficial (those you can see) core muscles with specific exercises to build strength, endurance, and flexibility.

Balance exercises that use the BOSU or exercise ball or yoga and Pilates classes are other options in developing your core. Remember your core is developed from the inner muscles to the outer. You should keep your core engaged not only during specific exercises but during all movements, including activities of daily living, walking, and sitting in an office chair.

### SUCCESS CHECK

☒ Choose a core exercise for each muscle group in the core that suits your fitness level.

☒ List at least one progression for each of your core exercises.

# CORE SUMMARY

The core is one of the most important muscle groups in your body. It supports you in every movement you make throughout the day. Make sure you are taking the time to strengthen and stretch all the muscles involved, not just the outer, visible portion. Remember also that the core can be engaged throughout the day, not just during workouts.

### Before Taking the Next Step

1. Are you able to stabilize your core performing the cat–cow exercise?

2. Did you choose one core exercise or sequence for each core muscle group to add to your fitness program?

3. Did you list the days and times of the week you will be incorporating core stability and mobility into your fitness routine?

# Nutrition

Exercise and healthy eating go hand in hand. Your overall health is affected by the foods you choose to eat every day. Nutrition is the process of consuming the food you need for health and growth because your body breaks down and rebuilds cells 24/7. So every morsel of food you put in your mouth either helps or hinders your health.

Proper nutrition along with exercise not only keeps your body strong and healthy but also helps prevent diseases such as obesity, diabetes, certain cancers, and heart disease. Healthy eating can also boost your immune system and ward off fatigue. It can delay the effects of aging, help you maintain your weight, and give you energy. Finally, eating well protects your bones and teeth and enhances your ability to concentrate and improve sport performance.

Whether you are trying to lose weight, gain muscle, or maintain your current fitness level, the most important part in the equation is nutrition. It doesn't matter how hard or how long your workout sessions are; without proper nutrition in the proper amounts, your body will not change, or it will change very slowly. The hard work you put in with exercise may be wasted because your body may resort to burning muscle (which slows metabolism) and storing fat.

## NUTRIENTS FOR OPTIMAL HEALTH

You have already learned the importance of exercise, and this step will help you understand the importance of your nutrition needs and how to meet those needs. A nutrient is a substance the body needs in order to work properly. The three macronutrients are protein, carbohydrate, and fat; the three micronutrients are minerals, vitamins, and water. All of these are needed for proper growth and functioning.

### Protein

Protein repairs and maintains the body. Protein is in every human body cell, and it is a major part of muscles, organs, skin, and glands. It is responsible for healthy blood cells and strengthening the immune system.

Protein is made up of amino acids; 20 amino acids combine to make all types of protein. There are 11 nonessential amino acids that your body can produce and 9 essential amino acids you must obtain from your diet. The protein that you eat is labeled according to the number of essential amino acids it provides.

A complete protein contains all of the essential amino acids and comes from animal sources such as fish, meat, poultry, eggs, milk, and cheese. Here are examples of protein:

- 3 ounces of meat (85 g) has 21 grams of protein
- 8 ounces of milk (240 ml) has 8 grams of protein
- 1 cup dry beans has 16 grams of protein

An incomplete protein is lacking one or more of the essential amino acids. Complementary proteins are two or more incomplete proteins that, when combined, provide adequate amounts of essential amino acids. This is particularly important if you are a vegetarian. Here are examples:

- Grains with legumes such as beans and rice; corn and beans; vegetarian chili with bread
- Grains and nuts and seeds such as peanut butter on whole-grain bread; breadstick with sesame seeds; rice with sesame seeds
- Legumes and nuts and seeds such as hummus and trail mix

How much protein to consume in a day depends on your activity level, muscle mass, health, and age. The average adult needs approximately 10 to 35 percent of daily food intake to be protein, which, according to the USDA, is about 46 grams for women and 56 grams for men. That is about 2 or 3 servings of protein daily. Too much protein can be a factor in high cholesterol and gout and can strain the kidneys. It's also important to know that eating excessive protein does not build more muscle or make you stronger. Excessive protein intake also contributes to weight gain. A healthy, balanced diet should provide enough protein without the need for supplements. However, certain people have a greater need for protein: pregnant (10 grams more) and lactating (20 grams more) women, athletes, bodybuilders, and very active people (about 50 percent more protein).

### SUCCESS CHECK

- ☒ What does protein do in the body?
- ☒ List two types of protein (or combinations) that you could eat for each meal: breakfast, lunch, and dinner.

# CARBOHYDRATE

Carbohydrate is made up of carbon, hydrogen, and oxygen and is the primary energy source used by the body. However, over the past several years fad diets have rated carbohydrate as a feared food. But research has shown that carbohydrate is instrumental in lowering the risk of chronic diseases. What are we to believe? Both claims are true, because there is good carbohydrate and bad carbohydrate.

Complex carbohydrate contains the sugar, fiber, and starch that help your body function properly. Although both complex and simple carbohydrates are broken down into sugar, complex carbohydrate contains fiber, which is the plant part that the body can't absorb or digest. When you eat high-fiber foods, the sugar is controlled and released slowly so your body can use the carbohydrate as fuel. In addition, less is stored as fat and your blood sugar remains stable. Fiber helps you avoid the spikes in blood sugar so you have energy to burn all day. Certain types of fiber, such as that found in oats, can lower cholesterol. Fiber can also aid in weight control by making you feel full and satisfied. Good carbohydrate can also reduce the risk of heart disease and colon cancer.

Carbohydrate helps the body absorb calcium, manage digestion by providing nutrients in the intestinal tract that help the good bacteria, and regulate the amount of sugar in the bloodstream. It is responsible for managing heart rate, breathing, and brain functioning. Once the body has used the carbohydrate it needs, some of the excess is stored as glycogen in the liver and muscles for energy, and the remainder is stored as fat.

One of the most important meals of the day is after a workout, where your muscles have a window for storing muscle glycogen for your next workout day. Make sure you eat a complex carbohydrate within that 30-minute window after a workout. On that same note, your body needs protein within an hour after a workout so muscle tissue can recover faster. One of the best postworkout foods is chocolate milk because it contains both carbohydrate and protein.

Simple carbohydrate, which is high in calories, includes processed grains that have had the fiber stripped away, such as the refined white grain and refined sugar. When you eat these foods, they start a cycle: They digest quickly and cause a sugar rush (a spike in your blood sugar level), then leave you fatigued, hungry, and craving more sugar. Don't forget that through this cycle your body is storing the excess carbohydrate as fat.

Foods that contain complex carbohydrate with fiber are whole grains, vegetables, fruits, and legumes. Here are examples of complex carbohydrate:

- **Whole grains:** brown rice, corn, wheat, barley, oats, spelt
- **Vegetables:** carrots, zucchini, cucumbers, radishes, asparagus, onions, spinach, broccoli, green beans, yams, potatoes
- **Fruits:** tomatoes, apples, pears, strawberries, grapefruit, peaches, cherries, bananas, plums, melons
- **Legumes:** peas, kidney beans, pinto beans, black beans, chickpeas, split peas, lentils

Examples of foods that are in the simple bad carb category are white bread, white pasta, sugary cereals, fruit juices, soft drinks, doughnuts, candy, cookies, and cake.

According to the USDA, adults need 45 to 65 percent of daily caloric intake from carbohydrate. That is about 130-190 grams of carbohydrate per day—your brain alone needs 100 grams of carbohydrate per day to function! Try to get at least 5 servings of fruits and vegetables per day.

### SUCCESS CHECK

- ☒ What does carbohydrate do in the body?
- ☒ List two examples of carbohydrate foods that you could eat for each meal: breakfast, lunch, and dinner.

# FAT

Like carbohydrate, fat has gotten a bad name recently as being unhealthy. People eliminate fat from their diets because they believe eating fat will make them fat. Any excess of fat, protein, or carbohydrate will end up being converted and stored as fat tissue; it's just that fat itself is easiest to store. Protein and carbohydrate must undergo several steps and processing to be stored. Stored fat is reserved energy (1 gram of fat contains 9 calories), but fat is responsible for many other important functions of the body. Fat helps other nutrients do their job. Without ingesting fat, your body can't absorb or transport the fat-soluble vitamins A, D, E, and K. Want healthy hair and skin? You must eat fat. Fat is responsible for brain development and healthy nerve functioning, control of inflammation, and clotting of the blood. It is also needed for hormone production.

The three types of dietary fat are saturated, unsaturated, and trans. Saturated fat is solid at room temperature and can cause high levels of LDL (bad) cholesterol. In addition, excessive saturated fat increases your risk of heart disease. Unsaturated fat is liquid at room temperature and healthier for you—it lowers your risk for heart disease. It helps you manage your mood and fight fatigue. Unsaturated fat is divided into two categories: polyunsaturated and monounsaturated. Omega-3 fat is a special type of polyunsaturated fat that research has declared especially beneficial because it can protect against memory loss and dementia, strengthen a healthy pregnancy, and reduce and even prevent depression. It also can ease joint pain and arthritis. In addition, this particular type of fat can reduce the risk of not only heart disease but also stroke and cancer.

Trans fat is produced by adding hydrogen to vegetable oil in a process called hydrogenation. It gives food a longer shelf life. Foods that include hydrogenated and partially hydrogenated oils not only can increase LDL (bad) cholesterol but also lower HDL (good cholesterol). In 2013 the FDA announced a proposal that would ban partially hydrogenated oil for use in food because research has indicated that trans fat is no longer safe to use in food. This affects how food is prepared not only in the fast food industry but also in the manufacturing of microwave popcorn, frozen pizza and desserts, baking mixes, cookies, and margarines, just to name a few.

Saturated fat is found in animal (beef, pork) and whole-fat dairy products (cheese, butter, whole milk, cream). Unsaturated fat is found in fish and most vegetable oils (olive, corn, canola, sunflower, safflower). You can also find good fat in avocados, nuts, seeds (sunflower, sesame, pumpkin, flaxseed), fatty fish (salmon, tuna, trout, sardines), soy milk, and tofu. Trans fat is found in processed foods (packaged foods such as crackers and chips) and commercial baked goods (cookies, doughnuts, cakes, pastries, fried foods, candy, and margarine).

According to the USDA, adults need 10 to 25 percent of their daily caloric intake from fat. That is about 30-40 grams of fat per day. However, the fat you eat needs to be good fat. Following are suggestions on substituting unsaturated fat for saturated fat:

- Bake or grill; don't fry.
- Choose lower-fat cheese and milk.
- Take the skin off of chicken.
- Avoid breaded vegetables and meat.
- Choose lean cuts of beef.
- Eat less red meat and more white meat and fish.
- Eat omega-3 fat in your diet every day: fish, walnuts, flaxseeds, canola oil.
- Cook with olive oil.
- Snack on nuts.
- Eliminate trans fat from your diet.

### SUCCESS CHECK

- ☒ What does fat do in the body?
- ☒ Distinguish between saturated fat and unsaturated fat.
- ☒ What are three sources of omega-3 fat?
- ☒ List two examples of fat foods that you could eat for each meal: breakfast, lunch, and dinner.

# WATER

Water is a nutrient essential for life—it's in every cell of your body. Your body is made up of 60 percent water: Body fat is 10 percent water, your brain is 85 percent water, muscles have 75 percent water, bones have 22 percent water, and blood contains 70 percent water. Every tissue and organ in your body contains water.

Your body needs water to maintain body temperature and uses water to get rid of waste products through perspiration, urination, and bowel movements. Water cushions and lubricates the joints and protects the spinal cord. It carries nutrients to the cells and helps you digest your food. Water is needed to absorb certain hormones and gives the muscles their natural ability to contract and maintain muscle tone. Water is important for maintaining great skin—it helps prevent sagging skin that follows extreme weight loss, and it softens the skin and reduces wrinkles.

Although you get about 80 percent of the water you need through the drinks you consume during the day, the remaining 20 percent comes from the foods you eat. Plain water is the best way to rehydrate your body, period. However, if you are an endurance athlete and spend hours exercising and sweating profusely, you may need to replace more than just water because your body loses electrolytes (calcium, sodium, magnesium, and potassium) that are essential in regulating nerves and muscles. If you don't like the sugary sport drinks, you have the option of consuming a healthier alternative by drinking water with a banana, raisins, dried figs, or chocolate milk. Or you can dilute the sport drink with 50 percent water.

Regardless of what the advertisements for sport drinks tell you, if your workout sessions are an hour or less, you don't need the same type of hydration with electrolytes as endurance athletes do. Sport drinks may replace the calories you just burned or add more calories that will be stored as fat. What about zero-calorie drinks that contain artificial sweeteners? The truth about artificial sweeteners through scientific research is discussed later in this step.

You have heard or read that you must drink 8 glasses of water a day. However, that is not completely true. The amount of water you need depends on several factors, including your age, activity, and environment. To stay hydrated, you need to drink enough water to replace the water you lost. Besides losing water every day through respiration, perspiration, urination and defecation, you lose water in hot weather and humidity; when you have a fever, vomiting, or diarrhea; or when you physically exert yourself working or exercising. You need enough water to make your urine pale yellow or clear—the easiest way to know if you are drinking enough water. If you wait until you are thirsty, your body is already dehydrated.

When exercising or participating in sports, you should drink 8 ounces (~240 ml) before, 4 ounces (~120 ml) every 15 minutes during, and 16 ounces (~480 ml) on completion of your workout. You will need more or less depending on the environment. If it is hot and humid, or you sweat profusely, you will need more water. Why not one of the sport drinks? Two reasons: First, your body begins to absorb water as soon as it hits your mouth, whereas other drinks must be digested. Second, many sport drinks contain excess calories that can wreak havoc on your diet.

Remember to stay clear of caffeinated drinks—they dehydrate, not hydrate, your body. If you are not currently consuming adequate amounts of water, here are some tips to help you increase your water intake:

- Keep a water bottle with you at all times.
- Choose water instead of soda, tea, or juice when eating out.
- Drink water before each meal.
- Add lemon, lime, or a few slices of cucumber to your water.
- Drink decaffeinated herbal tea or coffee instead of caffeinated.

# VITAMINS AND MINERALS

There are 13 vitamins our bodies needed to sustain life, and these organic compounds are essential for metabolism and crucial for health. If you don't get enough vitamins in your diet, it may cause deficiency diseases.

## Vitamins

The two types of vitamins are water soluble and fat soluble. Water-soluble vitamins are not stored for very long in the body, so they need to be replaced on a daily basis. Vitamin C and all the B-vitamins (called B-complex vitamins) are water soluble, and many times the vitamins are destroyed or washed out during food preparation and storage. Make sure fresh produce is refrigerated and milk and grains are stored away from light. Use the water from cooking vegetables in soup, which contains many of the vitamins lost to cooking.

The B-complex vitamins (thiamin, riboflavin, niacin, $B_6$, folate, $B_{12}$, biotin, and pantothenic acid) help the body get energy from food and are responsible for vision, appetite, healthy skin, red blood cells, and the nervous system. Fat-soluble vitamins are A, D, E, and K. These are stored in the liver and fat tissue for days and months. The body needs small amounts of these vitamins and doesn't need them every day, which means large amounts of these vitamins can be toxic and cause health problems. These vitamins dissolve in fat before the blood carries them through the body. Fat-soluble vitamins are responsible for these processes:

- Bone growth and tooth development
- Keeping mucous membranes moist (mouth, nose, lungs, throat)
- Antioxidants in preventing certain cancers
- Regulating the immune system
- Absorbing calcium
- Normal blood clotting

## Minerals

A well-balanced diet that includes a variety of foods is the best way to get all the vitamins and minerals your body needs. Fresh fruits and vegetables, whole grains, low-fat dairy, and poultry, fish, and lean red meat are the best choices for getting not only the vitamins and minerals you need but also protein, carbohydrate, and fat. Vitamin supplements are not recommended unless you are pregnant, are over age 50, or have a medical condition that affects the absorption of these nutrients, such as food allergies or irritable bowel syndrome, or if you consume a low-calorie diet. Before taking any supplements, you should consult with a registered dietitian who can help you make the best choices.

# SERVING SIZE

It's important to choose the right foods, but learning how to choose the correct portion size is equally important. Having a visual idea of what a serving size is will be helpful in eating the amount of food that your body needs.

According to the USDA, adults should consume 2 or 3 servings of protein per day. The protein should be lean or low-fat meat and poultry and seafood rich in omega-3 fatty acids. Include at least two servings per week of fish such as salmon, sardines, or trout. Limit processed protein as in packaged deli meats, hot dogs, sausage, and ham because of their high sodium content.

You need to include 6 to 11 servings of carbohydrate per day; at least 3-6 ounces of grain, half of which should be whole grain, 2-3 servings of vegetables, and 2-3 servings of fruit. Look for the Whole Grain Stamp that the USDA recommends to ensure what you are eating is 100 percent whole grain. Consuming fat is important, and it is recommended that you get 2 or 3 servings of fat per day. These servings should be unsaturated fat such as olive oil, walnuts, and seeds.

Of course you can measure each ounce or morsel of food, but an easier way is to visualize the amount of food in comparison to your hand. Following are examples of serving sizes (figure 9.1) that you can estimate when filling your plate:

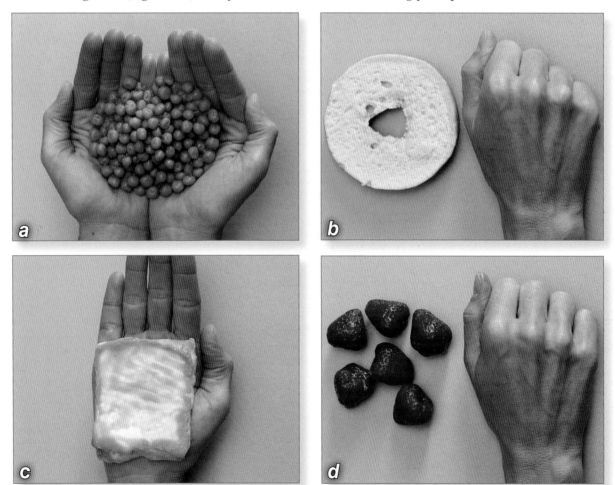

**Figure 9.1**   One serving of vegetables is what fits in the palms of both hands (*a*). One serving of grains (*b*) is about the size of your fist. One serving of meat should be able to fit in the palm of one hand (*c*). One serving of fruit is about the size of your fist (*d*).

*(continued)*

**Figure 9.1** *(continued)*

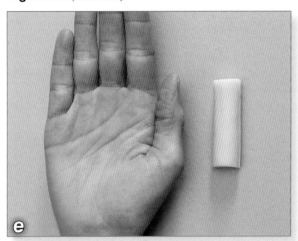

**Figure 9.1** One serving of dairy is as long as your thumb (*e*).

In addition to using your hand as a guide, the USDA has designed MyPlate, shown in figure 9.2, which will help you recognize not only portion size but also food choices for a healthy body. This is an excellent food tracker that can help you with healthy eating. For more information, go to www.choosemyplate.gov.

## SUCCESS CHECK

- ☒ List at least one serving of protein, carbohydrate, and fat that you can eat for each meal: breakfast, lunch, and dinner.
- ☒ Using your hand as a guide, demonstrate the portion size of protein, fruit, grains, vegetables, and dairy.

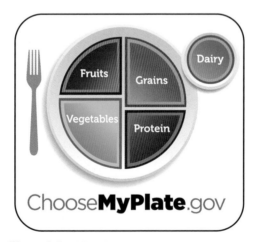

**Figure 9.2** My plate.

Source: USDA Center for Nutrition Policy and Promotion.

# FOOD LABELS

The can in the grocery store says "tuna in water." However, the list of ingredients says tuna, water, soy, carrots, and celery! In 1990 the Nutrition Labeling and Education Act was passed, and the USDA and FDA were in charge of deciding what information you need to know about the food you eat. Every food and beverage product must contain the following information:

- Nutrition facts are quantities of protein, fat (saturated, unsaturated, and trans), carbohydrate (sugar and fiber), vitamins, and minerals for one serving.
- Ingredients are contents listed in descending order.
- Serving size is what constitutes one serving.
- Product name.
- Manufacturer's name and address.
- Weight, measure, or count of the product.

Finding out whether a food product is healthy for you may be more difficult if you don't understand the product's label. Many times the claims on the front of the package are deceptive because they are not monitored as closely as the nutrition label on the back and may be misleading. You will see "fat-free," "no added sugar," "natural," "lite," and "helps your immune system" on labels to entice you to purchase the food item, but it's not clear what these labels really mean. We'll take a closer look at what some of these claims mean (per serving) so you will be better informed when you are pushing that cart through the market. See figure 9.3 on page 201 for a sample food label.

## Fat-Free, Sugar-Free, Zero Calories

This may be one of the most misleading topics because many people think that if a food is fat free or sugar free, it's healthy. If a food item has this label, the fat and sugar must be less than 0.5 gram per serving, and calorie free must be no more than 5 calories per serving. It's important to understand that just because a food item is fat free it may be very high in sugar and calories. If it claims to be sugar free, it still may be in high in fat and calories. Look at the total calories per serving to decide whether the food is healthy for your diet plan.

## Low Fat, Low Sugar, Low Calorie

This type of label on a product means it contains less than 3 grams of fat and less than 1 gram of saturated fat per serving. To be considered low calorie, the food must contain fewer than 40 calories per serving. This is where the manufacturer's front label can be deceiving, because the claim will be "no trans fat" on the front, but the actual nutrition label may indicate that saturated or unsaturated fat content is high, and may legally contain up to 0.5 gram of trans fat. If you eat more than one serving of this "no-trans-fat" food, the trans fat can add up.

## Natural

Not surprisingly, this label has no real definition and it can be whatever the manufacturer wants it to be! According to the FDA, as long as the product has no artificial flavors, added color, or synthetic substances, it can be called natural. Foods such as yogurt, granola bars, nondairy cheese, and honey that you thought were healthy may not be. The purple color and flavor in yogurt may not be from blueberries! And the 100 percent natural jar of honey you just bought home isn't technically honey due to so many levels of processing that removes the natural pollen. Purchase honey from a local beekeeper or at a farmer's market for truly natural honey.

What about the granola bar—the staple of many fitness fanatics for a snack or after-workout food? Many of these bars, sometimes called energy bars or protein bars, contain an ingredient made from wood pulp or cotton (called cellulose) to up the fiber content. They also contain processed sweeteners. They may not be healthy for you at all! Make sure you read not only the nutrition label but the ingredients as well.

## Organic

A food labeled as organic is not the same as being 100 percent natural. If a food is labeled as organic, it must pass specific USDA guidelines, which state that animal products must not have antibiotics or growth hormones, and plants must be grown without the use of pesticides or synthetic fertilizers. You will notice that the levels of organic range from 70 to 100 percent, depending on how they were grown.

## Fresh

This label means not only that the food must be unprocessed or raw, but that it has never been heated or frozen. Although this may sound like a great food source, this label doesn't mean the food was just picked. You never know how long it has been in transit to the store or how long it has been sitting on the shelf. This may increase the surface bacteria on these foods, so make sure you wash all fresh foods before preparing or eating them.

You can use a nutrition label to help you choose foods that are healthy for your body. Don't simply look at the total grams of carbohydrate in foods; rather, choose those that are high in fiber and low in sugar. See what type of fat (unsaturated, saturated, or trans fat) is in the food.

Look at the list of ingredients to see if sugar or fat is one of the first four ingredients listed. If so, this food probably is not the best choice. Also look for sugar alcohols, which are actually neither sugar nor alcohol but a chemical structure that sweetens food and can cause intestinal problems. Sugar alcohols usually end in —ol, such as sorbitol and mannitol.

### SUCCESS CHECK

☒ Name three ways food labels can help you choose a healthy food product.

☒ What type of fat should you avoid when purchasing a food product?

# METABOLISM

Metabolism is the rate at which the body burns calories. Several factors affect metabolic rate: sex, body size, age, activity level, the environment, muscle mass, genetics, and the thermic effect of food. First you must understand that basal metabolic rate is the amount of calories needed to sustain life—breathing, blood flow, and body

Check the serving size and number of servings.

- The Nutrition Facts label information is based on ONE serving, but many packages contain more. Look at the serving size and how many servings you are actually consuming. If you double the servings you eat, you double the calories and nutrients, including the % DVs.
- When you compare calories and nutrients between brands, check to see if the serving size is the same.

Calories count, so pay attention to the amount.

- This is where you'll find the number of calories per serving and the calories from fat in each serving.
- Fat-free doesn't mean calorie-free. Lower fat items may have as many calories as full-fat versions.
- If the label lists that 1 serving equals 3 cookies and 100 calories, and you eat 6 cookies, you've eaten 2 servings, or twice the number of calories and fat.

Look for foods that are rich in these nutrients.

- Use the label not only to limit fat and sodium, but also to increase nutrients that promote good health and may protect you from disease.
- Some Americans don't get enough vitamins A and C, potassium, calcium, and iron, so choose the brand with the higher % DV for these nutrients.
- Get the most nutrition for your calories—compare the calories to the nutrients you would be getting to make a healthier food choice.

# Nutrition Facts

Serving Size 1 cup (228g)
Servings Per Container 2

**Amount Per Serving**

**Calories** 250     Calories from Fat 110

| | % Daily Value* |
|---|---|
| **Total Fat** 12g | 18% |
| Saturated Fat 3g | 15% |
| *Trans* Fat 3g | |
| **Cholesterol** 30mg | 10% |
| **Sodium** 470mg | 20% |
| **Potassium** 700mg | 20% |
| **Total Carbohydrate** 31g | 10% |
| Dietary Fiber 0g | 0% |
| Sugars 5g | |
| **Protein** 5g | |

| | |
|---|---|
| Vitamin A | 4% |
| Vitamin C | 2% |
| Calcium | 20% |
| Iron | 4% |

* Percent Daily Values are based on a 2,000 calorie diet. Your Daily Values may be higher or lower depending on your calorie needs.

| | Calories: | 2,000 | 2,500 |
|---|---|---|---|
| Total fat | Less than | 65g | 80g |
| Sat fat | Less than | 20g | 25g |
| Cholesterol | Less than | 300mg | 300mg |
| Sodium | Less than | 2,400mg | 2,400mg |
| Total Carbohydrate | | 300g | 375g |
| Dietary Fiber | | 25g | 30g |

The % Daily Value is a key to a balanced diet.

The % DV is a general guide to help you link nutrients in a serving of food to their contribution to your total daily diet. It can help you determine if a food is high or low in a nutrient—5% or less is low, 20% or more is high. You can use the % DV to make dietary trade-offs with other foods throughout the day. The * is a reminder that the % DV is based on a 2,000-calorie diet. You may need more or less, but the % DV is still a helpful gauge.

Know your fats and reduce sodium for health.

- To help reduce your risk of heart disease, use the label to select foods that are lowest in saturated fat, *trans* fat, and cholesterol.
- *Trans* fat doesn't have a % DV, but consume as little as possible because it increases your risk of heart disease.
- The % DV for total fat includes all different kinds of fats.
- To help lower blood cholesterol, replace saturated and *trans* fats with monounsaturated and polyunsaturated fats found in fish, nuts, and liquid vegetable oils.
- Limit sodium to help reduce your risk of high blood pressure.

For protein, choose foods that are lower in fat.

- Most Americans get plenty of protein, but not always from the healthiest sources.
- When choosing a food for its protein content, such as meat, poultry, dry beans, milk and milk products, make choices that are lean, low-fat, or fat free.

Reach for healthy, wholesome carbohydrates.

- Fiber and sugars are types of carbohydrates. Healthy sources, like fruits, vegetables, beans, and whole grains, can reduce the risk of heart disease and improve digestive functioning.
- Whole grain foods can't always be identified by color or name, such as multi-grain or wheat. Look for the "whole" grain listed first in the ingredient list, such as whole wheat, brown rice, or whole oats.
- There isn't a % DV for sugar, but you can compare the sugar content in grams among products.
- Limit foods with added sugars (sucrose, glucose, fructose, corn or maple syrup), which add calories but not other nutrients, such as vitamins and minerals. Make sure that added sugars are not one of the first few items in the ingredients list.

**Figure 9.3** How to read a food label.

temperature—and amounts to approximately 1,200 calories for women and 1,500 calories for men per day. Resting metabolic rate is about 10 percent higher and includes not only breathing, blood flow, and body temperature but also energy used during daily activities and the thermic effect of food.

Men have a higher metabolism than women because of larger muscle mass. That's why men tend to lose fat at a faster rate than women. Metabolism slows down with age, but you can make adjustments by increasing your activity or reducing caloric intake to ward off the added pounds. Remember that muscle is active tissue, so the more muscle mass you gain, the higher your metabolism will be. Muscle increases the rate at which you burn calories 24/7!

As you strive to become fit, make sure you are eating a sufficient amount of calories. Not eating enough or going on a crash diets slows your metabolism and tends to store fat that you may be trying to burn. Also, your metabolism will be higher if you are in an environment that is hot or cold, and it may be higher due to a genetic disposition. Finally, the thermic effect of food increases metabolism. Yes, eating will help you burn fat! The thermic effect of food is energy used to digest, absorb, and distribute the nutrients in the food. Each time you eat, your body flips on a switch that stays on two to three house after you eat. If you choose to eat five or six small meals (breakfast, snack, lunch, snack, dinner), you will have the thermic effect of food longer throughout the day than if you choose to skip breakfast or eat only two or three times per day. Also, eating five or six small meals, which is about every 2.5 to 3 waking hours, keeps blood sugar and appetite hormones stabilized.

### SUCCESS CHECK

- ☒ How can you increase your metabolism?
- ☒ Why is it better to eat five or six small meals rather than two or three bigger meals per day?

# SUPPLEMENTS

You wander through the health food store and observe containers that promise muscle gain or fat loss or exercise in a bottle. Supplements are a hot topic today, and manufacturers are raking in over $5 billion a year in herbal supplements alone!

A supplement is something that completes or enhances something else when added to your diet. The FDA does not regulate or analyze supplements because supplements are not considered a food or a drug. The responsibility falls to the manufacturer to ensure the product is safe. Supplements don't have to be tested or proven safe before showing up on the shelf of the pharmacy, grocery store, or health food store. You will notice the label on supplements is similar to the Nutrition Facts label on food items, but it says Supplement Facts. You will also notice that when manufacturers make specific claims on a label, they are required by law to include a disclaimer stating that this claim has not been FDA approved. Only through consumer complaints does the FDA take action to investigate and test a supplement, such as when the supplement ephedra was finally banned because it was dangerous to consumers. Even then, it took several years to get the product off the shelf, and it's still available in herbal "all-natural" forms.

Supplements don't always contain the ingredients the label specifies, and they could also contain additives that are not listed in the ingredients at all. Several studies have uncovered some alarming practices, including the use of toxic ingredients not mentioned in ingredients lists and products that contain none of the ingredients listed. Many herbal supplements test positive for lead, mercury, arsenic, and pesticides—all hazardous substances.

Protein powder is a popular supplement that comes in various forms such as whey, soy, and casein. These supplements also vary in price. Sometimes the cheaper ones sound like a better deal, but they may not contain the essential amino acids your body can't make on its own. Although most people get more than enough protein through diet (it takes only 10 to 14 extra grams of protein per day to build a pound of muscle), there are very special situations where you may need to add protein. Always check with your doctor and registered dietitian first. Following are some special populations and situations that require additional protein:

- Growing teenagers
- Beginning weight trainers
- Longer workouts (going from 30-minute workouts to training for a triathlon)
- Injury recovery
- Vegetarians

Supplements can take up the slack in your diet when you are not getting enough of the nutrients you need. For example, bone density has been shown to increase for postmenopausal women when they consumed calcium and vitamin D supplements. However, getting what your body needs through real food is the best way to optimize your health. Researching the product, seeing your doctor, and engaging the help of a registered dietitian (RD) are your best defense in choosing not only what your body needs but also what is safe, especially if you are taking medications. You also need to look for the USP Verified label, which means the manufacturers had the product tested for safety.

### SUCCESS CHECK

- ☒ How can you determine whether a supplement is safe?
- ☒ Name three instances when you may need a supplement in your diet

# NUTRITION SUMMARY

Remember that food is fuel for your body, just as gas is for an automobile. You must put fuel in your car (body) at the beginning of a trip (breakfast) and stop periodically to refuel (lunch, dinner, and snacks.) When you reach your destination (end of the day), you park your car in the garage and no additional fuel is needed. Take a look at your current diet and find out where you need to make some changes to make better choices, increase intake of specific nutrients, or decrease intake of unhealthy foods. And don't forget to use the free USDA website for nutrition and tracking information: www.choosemyplate.gov.

## Before Taking the Next Step

1. Do you know how many servings of protein, carbohydrate, and fat your body needs each day?

2. Can you demonstrate serving sizes using your hand as a guide?

3. Can you list ways to increase water intake throughout the day?

4. Do you know how to read a food label?

5. Do you know what nutrients your body needs before and after workouts?

6. Have you listed the food choices for your meals and snacks?

# Behavior Change

You've been there—trying to change a behavior whether it is starting something new such as healthy eating or beginning an exercise program. Or you've tried to stop an unhealthy behavior such as smoking, eating unhealthy foods, or being a couch potato. You probably tried to do it on will power and probably failed more than once. Or you may be pretty good at eating healthy throughout the day but then blow it when you get home in front of the TV. How can you not only change your behavior but also have the new behavior become part of your lifestyle?

You must first understand the stages of change and where you stand. Then you will learn strategies for changing behaviors and how to put these strategies into practice. It's not an easy journey, but the time and effort you put into changing your behavior will be well worth it in the end.

## READINESS TO CHANGE

You may desperately want to lose weight or run your first 5K race, but are you ready? Can you commit to finding out how you can begin eating healthy and exercising regularly? There are five stages of change, and recognizing which stage you are in will help you be successful in moving into the next stage in reaching your health and fitness goals.

### Precontemplation Stage

If you are in this stage, you have no intention of starting any healthy behavior within the next 6 months. You believe you have no problem or believe that you have no control over your problem. You may be in denial or you may be ignoring the problem completely, and you're just not ready to make a change. Do any of these comments describe your thinking?

- I'm really not overweight; I'm just big boned.
- I can't exercise because I have bad knees.
- I've been fat all my life. It's in my genes.
- I don't need to do cardiorespiratory exercise because I'm not overweight.

If you recognize that you are in the precontemplation stage, you are encouraged to learn the risks of your behavior. You can start by asking questions such as these: What happens to your health when you are overweight? What happens to your heart if you don't exercise? How do genes affect your body composition? You need to perform a self-analysis in this stage.

## Contemplation Stage

If you're in this stage, you are aware that it would be beneficial to make a change, but you identify barriers to avoid doing so. Most people are in this stage, and it can last for months or years. You may have conflicting feelings thinking you have to give something up instead of thinking you're gaining something beneficial, so you keep putting it off. In this stage you are getting ready to make a change within the next 6 months. Can you relate to any of the following comments?

- I would feel better if I exercised, but I don't have time.
- Preparing meals instead of buying fast food would be cheaper and healthier, but I hate to grocery shop and cook, plus I don't have time.
- Paying the monthly fee at the gym would leave less money in the budget for new clothes.
- I just started a new job, so I can't start an exercise program until I'm settled in.

If you are in the contemplation stage, it is helpful to weigh the pros and cons. Identify barriers that are keeping you from starting an exercise program or eating healthier, and ways you can eliminate these barriers.

## Preparation Stage

In this stage you get information about the changes you want to make and take small steps in moving forward; you're ready. Within the next month, you will be taking action.

- You purchase fitness shoes and clear your schedule to walk 30 minutes a day.
- You tell your family and friends you're going to lose weight.
- You find out the times at the gym for yoga and cycling classes.
- You make a grocery list of healthy foods to purchase and have on hand.

If you are in the preparation stage, you are preparing a plan of action, which may include writing down your goals or preparing time in your schedule to go to the gym.

## Action Stage

In the action stage, you take direct action. You have changed your behavior for the past 6 months by eating healthy and exercising, but you must work hard to continue on this path. You think about going back to your old ways on and off during this period. These 6 months are one of the most critical times for changing a behavior because lapses are very common in this stage, and you are undoubtedly at risk for a relapse.

- You are walking 30 minutes a day and involved in weight training twice a week.
- You are eating not only a variety of healthy foods but also the correct portion sizes.
- You have lost fat and gained lean muscle. Your waistline is getting smaller.

If you are in the action stage, you are congratulating yourself on each successful behavior change and reinforcing the steps you are taking in making this change. You may have specific motivating statements that fill your mind. You may have an exercise buddy who keeps you accountable and vice versa. You exercise and eat healthy for the external rewards.

## Maintenance Stage

If you are in the maintenance stage, you have passed the 6-month mark of healthy eating and exercise! You are motivated to continue the behavior and are avoiding the temptation to return to the old behavior. You foresee obstacles in your fitness journey (vacations, holidays, illness, family emergencies) and have a plan in place to remedy the situation you're in. If you lapse in one of your behaviors, you recognize you are not perfect and jump right back in to your fitness regimen—no beating yourself up anymore.

- Your daily exercise is as much a part of your lifestyle as brushing your teeth.
- You look forward to challenging your muscles and keeping them strong.
- You prefer to eat lean protein and greens for lunch instead of a hamburger and fries.
- You exercise and eat healthy for the internal rewards—how it makes you feel.

In this stage you have developed strategies for turning down temptations and reward yourself for success. These rewards are intrinsic—they come from within. You know how great you feel after a workout and have a sense of accomplishment; you are in full control of your fitness and healthy eating.

Although you may identify a stage you are in right now, you can move in and out of different stages depending on what is happening in your life. For example, you may be in the action stage where you have been exercising regularly for 2 months and then suffer an acute or chronic injury, such as shin splints. Or a new job has left you working overtime or traveling for the past month and you have reverted to eating fast food on the road. Recognizing the stages and knowing where you stand are important in learning how to change your behavior.

### *SUCCESS CHECK*

- ☒ Name the five stages of change.
- ☒ Identify your current stage.
- ☒ Describe your current stage.

# STEPS TO CHANGING BEHAVIOR

The first step in changing a behavior is recognizing the behavior you want to change. As in any journey, you need to know where you're going before you start. For instance, if you recognized that you are in the precontemplation stage and you want to move to the contemplation stage, you may want to use photos or educational materials to raise your consciousness of the unhealthy behavior in which you are involved. If you want to change your smoking behavior, an example is comparing pictures of healthy lungs to pictures of lungs exposed to cigarettes. This may get you ready to move into the contemplation stage. Or maybe you have been in the preparation stage, renewing your gym membership every year but not using the facility at all! Perhaps you have been exercising regularly in the action stage and then struggle when your schedule changes due to illness, work, or the holidays, and you completely stop your regular fitness routine.

The next step is learning everything you can about the new behavior you desire. As in any journey, you need to learn about traveling to your destination. For example, if you want to eat healthier, learn the variety of foods your body needs. If you want to lose weight, learn about portion size and the types of exercise that are needed. If you want to lose body fat or get stronger, you need to learn the types of exercise that will make this happen. This step involves weighing the costs of the behavior change against the benefits. Making time to exercise may require you to get up an hour earlier, or eating healthier may require you to learn how to cook healthier meals.

Finally, you are ready to design a plan for the behavior change. As with any journey, this will be your road map to success. Schedule the days of the week and the times you will be exercising. It may be that the exercise will be short bouts throughout the day or involve getting up earlier. Make a grocery list and prepare healthy foods for the week. Monitor your progress on a regular basis by writing down your workout information and doing a fitness assessment every 4 to 6 weeks. Keep a food diary of the foods you eat, what time of day you eat them, and how you are feeling. Engage in strategies to help you on this journey.

### SUCCESS CHECK

- ☒ Name the three steps in changing your behavior.
- ☒ List at least two things you can do in each step.

# STRATEGIES FOR CHANGING BEHAVIOR

It's important to develop strategies before setting on your fitness journey. Strategies are how you will achieve changing your behavior so you can reach your fitness goals. Not to be confused with action, which is the who-what-when, strategies take into account your current barriers and resources available to you. How are you going to exercise regularly instead of sporadically? How are you going to choose healthy options at the holiday event? Following are several ways to help you change your behavior and reach your fitness goals.

## Change One Behavior at a Time

Your unhealthy behavior didn't happen overnight, and a new behavior will take time. Remember you will not use will power in starting a new behavior or stopping an old behavior but will replace one unhealthy behavior with a healthy behavior. Trying to accomplish too much too fast may set you up for failure and cause you to lapse, which can lead to relapse. So focus on one thing at a time.

## Get Support

Tell a friend or family member about your desire to change a behavior. Or if you feel you need help in starting a fitness or healthy eating program, seek the services of a personal trainer, support group, or registered dietitian. You may need the weekly meeting or may only need to meet a few times periodically throughout your journey to keep you on track and make progress.

## Make a Realistic and Specific Plan

If you want to start exercising 60 minutes 7 days a week but have a tight schedule, you are setting yourself up to fail. Be realistic, and write the 3 days and times in your planner that fit best. It's more realistic and doable to write down when you can exercise 3 days a week for 30 minutes instead of 7 days a week for an hour. Or maybe you can squeeze in 10-minute walks throughout the day. Remember you can always increase the time or add another day as your schedule allows. This will allow you to pat yourself on the back for accomplishing more than planned instead of beating yourself up because you missed an exercise session.

## Start With Small, Short-Term Goals

Although you may have large, long-term goals, they need to be broken down into smaller, realistic steps. Your long-term goal may be to lose 25 pounds, but breaking that down into a smaller goal will help you feel successful and motivated to continue. Losing a pound a week is a small, achievable step that will help you reach your goal in 25 weeks. If your goal is to eat healthier, you can start by eating a piece of fruit or yogurt for dessert three or four times a week.

## Use the Buddy System

Find someone who will go to the gym with you or who has similar goals in healthy eating. Having someone to keep you accountable when you want to skip the gym will help keep you on track and vice versa. Your buddy will be someone you can share experiences with, which can help you stay motivated and focused on changing your behavior.

## Set Up Prompts

Setting up daily reminders, or prompts, will help you stay focused in changing your behavior. Pack your gym bag the night before, or keep your running shoes in the car. Put your exercise schedule on the refrigerator. Schedule your exercise time in your planner as you would a doctor's appointment. Have healthy to-go snacks with you throughout the day.

## Use Rewards

It's important to recognize your accomplishment! Upon reaching a specific behavior, reward yourself with a movie or spa treatment instead of an unhealthy food item. If your goal is to lose weight, celebrate the first 5 pounds lost. If you entered your first 5K race and crossed the finish line, treat yourself to something special. Use your social media network to post, tweet, or blog about what you have accomplished.

## Don't Get Bored

It's easy to get stuck in a rut when it comes to exercise and healthy eating. Think about changing your regular walking route, or vary your activity with walking, biking, or swimming. This is the time to try something new: Take a yoga class or sign up for martial arts lessons. If you have been doing the same strength routine, switch it up with 1 to 2 weeks of body-weight exercises. It's also good to try different recipes or foods you haven't tried before.

## Use Stimulus Control

If you are aware of certain triggers—or stimuli—that set off an unhealthy behavior, make a note of the time, place, and your feelings when it happens and choose an alternative. For example, if you drive by fast food on the way home and can't resist the fries or milkshake, take a different route—out of sight, out of mind! If certain people sabotage you with unhealthy behavior, avoid hanging out with them until you have the behavior under control. If you regularly meet for wings on Friday night, eat before you go. Can't resist sweets? Do not bring them into your home. If you have to get in your car and drive to the store to buy the sweets you are craving, you may realize it's not worth the bother.

## Monitor Your Behavior

Keep a record of your workouts regarding what type of exercise you performed. Did you do 30 minutes on the elliptical? Or 3 sets of exercises for your back and chest? How much weight and how many reps did you complete? Did you eat 5 fruits and vegetables today? Keep a written account of all the calories consumed in a day. Studies have shown that those who monitor their exercise lose more weight and increase fitness levels than those who don't. And those who keep track of their eating are more likely to choose healthy foods and correct portion sizes. Today's technology with smartphone apps and interactive websites make monitoring this information easier than in the past.

## Learn How to Be Positive

Being positive not only makes your brain more productive but also reduces stress. Many times unhealthy behavior such as smoking or indulging in chocolate is a mechanism people turn to when tired, hungry, or emotionally used up. You might use it to manage stress and anxiety, which results in creating additional negativity and guilt.

To be more positive, write down one good thing that happened to you in the past 24 hours and relive it. Take the opportunity when stuck in traffic or waiting on a red light to reflect on something you are grateful for. Find an image that always makes you smile and use it as a screensaver, or perform a random act of kindness. Most of all, turn off the negative self-talk, and turn on the tapes in your head with all the good qualities you have!

### SUCCESS CHECK

☒  List five strategies that help in changing a behavior.

# HOW LONG DOES IT TAKE TO CHANGE BEHAVIOR?

Everyone wants instant results. But research has proven that because each person is unique, it can take 3 weeks to almost a year to change a behavior. This is because actual physical changes occur in the brain during the behavior change process. These changes depend on several factors:

- How long you have had the unhealthy behavior. Have you been sedentary 3 years or 25 years?
- The frequency of the unhealthy behavior. Do you smoke only on the weekends, or is it a pack a day?
- The benefit of changing the behavior. Are you giving up the all-you-can-eat wings every Tuesday night with your friends to fit in your workout in for the day?

The new choices you will make need to occur over and over and be reinforced for many months before your brain rewires and establishes the new healthy behavior over the old unhealthy behavior. So instead of focusing on a deadline such as 30 days, 6 months, or a year as an event when the new you will be unveiled, concentrate on the daily process required to change the behavior. Get through one day at a time or even a half day at a time. Your new behavior will eventually add up to days, weeks, and months, which will give your brain time to rewire.

# STAYING MOTIVATED

You have more than likely experienced the motivation every January when people make resolutions to be more active and make healthier food choices. But what happens when February rolls around? Or maybe you are motivated to get in shape for your class reunion or a wedding, and after the event you revert to your previous unhealthy behavior. How can you stay motivated until your new behavior becomes your lifestyle?

First and foremost, the only person who can motivate you is you! Motivation is the desire and willingness to take action inside you, and it is different in each person. It can be strong or weak and can change throughout your life depending on your circumstances. And although others may influence or inspire you, you are the only person who can motivate yourself. No one else can make you do something you don't want to do.

Second, nobody is perfect and you need to realize that lapses are not only common but inevitable, so stop the all-or-nothing attitude. A lapse is a time for you to stop and learn what strategy didn't work for you and to develop a new strategy. Instead of focusing on what you did or didn't do that was unhealthy, focus on what you can do next time when you are in the same situation. Take it a day at a time.

# RELAPSE PREVENTION

Having a lapse means that you slipped up once or even a few times. When you have several lapses in behavior, it may lead to a relapse, which means you have reverted to your old unhealthy behavior. This is more common than you think. In a relapse, you may label yourself a failure and beat yourself up over frustration. Do any of the following sound familiar?

- You overdid it at the buffet and consumed a huge amount of unhealthy food. You then give yourself permission to eat unhealthy for the rest of the week because you already messed up.

- You missed a week of workouts due to the flu but stayed out of the gym for a month. Besides, the weather was cold and your favorite TV series is starting back up.

- You gained 8 pounds on your 2-week cruise in the Caribbean and realize it's going to be a struggle to lose the weight yet again. So you put off making the commitment you once had.

If you are in a relapse, first understand it is common. You may feel frustrated and disappointed in yourself, but it's important to know how to recover. The first thing you need to do is have a plan in place that will get you back on track. Studies have shown that in order to stay in the maintenance stage where healthy eating and exercise are your lifestyle, you must know what to do when you have a relapse.

First you need to identify what led to this behavior. Was it an event like an illness or a long vacation that got you off track? Maybe your schedule got too busy to include your regular routine. Recognize what happened that started the relapse.

Second, you need to learn how you can overcome it the next time it happens. Have a plan of action next time you plan to go to a buffet, get sick, or go away on vacation. For example, the next time you go to a buffet, use the one-plate rule: Fill one plate with as much as it can hold, and don't go back for seconds. Or when on vacation, have a plan to eat a healthy breakfast and lunch, then splurge on dinner. You won't feel deprived or disappointed.

Third, understand and realize that messing up one time does not make you a failure. It helps to remind yourself of all the hard work it took to get you to where you are and that you are not going to undo everything you have accomplished. Learn what you can change next time you are faced with the situation, whatever it may be.

Finally, get back on track immediately. Don't wait for Monday to roll around or wait until tomorrow. If you slip up in the afternoon and cave in to that candy bar, write it off and get back on track. Don't use it as an excuse to gorge yourself on sweets and unhealthy foods for the rest of the day. Continue to follow the healthy eating plan you made. If you missed a week of workouts due to the flu, know that your body composition is not going to change in one week, and plan to return as soon as you are able.

## SUCCESS CHECK

☒ List what to do when you have a lapse or relapse in behavior.

# BEHAVIOR CHANGE SUMMARY

Remember that fitness is a lifestyle, and it involves healthy eating and regular exercise. Getting fit doesn't happen overnight, and being successful and reaching goals have little to do with will power, but they involve making a behavior change.

Learning how to make a behavior change involves knowing where you stand, identifying triggers that cause you to lapse, and using strategies that can help keep you on track and stay motivated. Making a plan of action for the next 24 hours, the next week, or the next month will become a road map to success. Remember that the only person who can change you is you.

### Before Starting Your Journey

1. Did you identify your current stage of behavior?
2. Do you know the steps it takes to change your behavior?
3. List at least six strategies that will help you change your behavior.
4. Name three ways you can prevent a relapse from happening.

Fitness Assessment   #_____          Date _____

| Health Screen | | |
|---|---|---|
| Age | BP | Pulse |
| Weight | Height | Fat % |
| Fat lbs | LBM | BMI |

| Girth Measurements | |
|---|---|
| Shoulders | Chest |
| Waist | Hips |
| Thigh | Bicep |

| Posture | |
|---|---|
| Front View | Side View |
| Ears level | Chin parallel to floor |
| Shoulders level | Ear in line with shoulder |
| Hips level | Shoulders not rounded forward |
| Arms equal distance from sides | Chest up |
| Arms by side, palms facing front | Slight curve in upper back |
| Toes slightly pointed out | Knees over the ankles |

| Fitness Testing |
|---|

| Balance | | | |
|---|---|---|---|
| Right Leg | sec | Left Leg | sec |

| Wall-sit | |
|---|---|
| Results | Rating |

| Push-Up Test | |
|---|---|
| Results | Rating |

| Curl-Up Test | |
|---|---|
| Results | Rating |

| Cardio Test | |
|---|---|
| Results | Rating |

| Pass / Fail Flexibility Tests | | | | | |
|---|---|---|---|---|---|
| Neck Flexion | PASS | FAIL | Shoulder Mob. L | PASS | FAIL |
| Left Quad | PASS | FAIL | Shoulder Flex R | PASS | FAIL |
| Right Quad | PASS | FAIL | Shoulder Flex L | PASS | FAIL |
| Low Back | PASS | FAIL | Shoulder Abduc. R | PASS | FAIL |
| Right Hamstring | PASS | FAIL | Shoulder Abduc. L | PASS | FAIL |
| Left Hamstring | PASS | FAIL | Hip Flexor R | PASS | FAIL |
| Right Calf | PASS | FAIL | Hip Flexor L | PASS | FAIL |
| Left Calf | PASS | FAIL | Trunk Rotation R | PASS | FAIL |
| Shoulder Mob. R | PASS | FAIL | Trunk Rotation L | PASS | FAIL |

From N.L. Naternicola, 2015, *Fitness: Steps to success* (Champaign, IL: Human Kinetics).